KID SMART!
Raising a Healthy Child

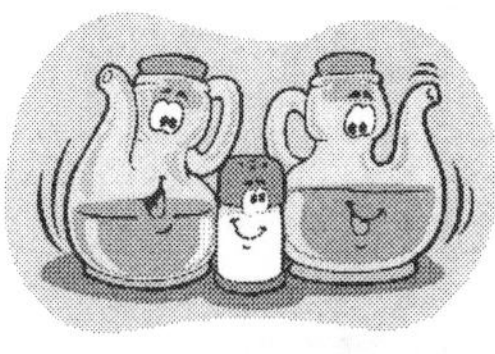

CHERYL TOWNSLEY

Lifestyle for Health Publishing
P.O. Box 3871, Littleton, CO 80161

ISBN 0-9644566-4-8

Graphics: Nick Zellinger
Cover Photo: Bill Peyton
Text Design: Theresa Frank

This publication is designed to provide accurate and authoritative information in regard to the subject matter covered. It is sold with the understanding that the author and the publisher are not engaged in rendering legal, medical, or other professional service. If medical services or other expert consultation is required, the services of a competent professional should be sought.

Townsley, Cheryl
Kid smart : raising a healthy child / Cheryl Townsley
Includes bibliographical references
ISBN 0-9644566-4-8
1. Health. 2. Nutrition. 3. Cookbook. I. Title.

For information contact:

Lifestyle for Health Publishing
P.O. Box 3871
Littleton, CO 80161
For ordering information, refer to the last page.

Printed in the United States of America

Contents

Part Three: Powerful Alternatives

Part Four: Resources

You made me a MOMMY!
You made Forest a DADDY!
You added a whole new dimension to our lives.
God has truly blessed us with a special bundle of joy...

That's you, ANNA.

We love you dearly and bless you with all of the health God created you to have.

Acknowledgments

Many people come together in order for a book to be born. The same is true for *Kid Smart!* I may have the inspiration, but the rest of the team help pull it together in a finished product you will want to read.

Thanks to Theresa Frank for hours of editing, typesetting and, text design. Each little detail on the written page came from T.F.'s mighty hands.

Thanks to Ed Hinckley for his knowledge and expertise. His editing and research were invaluable in our accuracy.

Thanks to Lory Floyd for once again adding her eagle-sharp eyes to our text. Her editing skills perfectly match my writing. She catches all of my errors.

Thanks to Marcia Pittleman for her research on the alternatives. Brands change ingredients and we wanted a completely current list of nutrients as of the printing of this book.

Thanks to Nick Zellinger for his creative cover design. His expertise with art, photos and computers make a professional transition from my kitchen to the world.

Thanks to Jerry Welch for the photo layout. Your creativity in our publishing and media adventures has been invaluable.

Thanks to Bill Peyton for his "art" in front of and behind the camera. He brings life to any photo. He is our favorite photographer.

Thanks to KIMCO for once again successfully bringing off the press a book that we hope will help America heal her children.

Thanks to Valerie Holmes for her consistent, professional help in booking media and personal appearances. Her welcoming voice and prompt follow-up bring a high level of customer service to our Lifestyle for Health customers.

Last, but absolutely not least, thanks to Forest and Anna for all of your prayers and support during a book-writing adventure. I am blessed to have you as my family.

All of these people are dear friends as well as professional co-workers. Working with people who are pros and enjoyable as people provides a great working environment. More creativity is released because of such unity and mutual respect. To you I say, "Thanks! And May God return a hundredfold to you in that which money can and cannot buy for your unselfish giving!"

Cheryl Townsley

—☆—

Introduction

As I watch adults and children go through the check-out lane at grocery stores, I am continually amazed and aghast at the contents of their carts. Their carts are piled high with packaged foods, sugared snacks and sodas, and many other non-food items. Occasionally I will see a head of iceberg lettuce or a few bananas peeping over the piles of "other stuff." I look from the cart to the child and then to the adult. The face of such food choices is always apparent.

Today we see more overweight children, more life-threatening diseases (such as heart disease, cancer, and leukemia) striking at younger and younger ages, and an increased onslaught of behavior and emotional problems manifesting through ADD. *Why?* The primary reasons are that our children are eating the Standard American Diet (SAD), rich in fast food, and are exposed to more and more toxins. We are experiencing a generational pattern of destruction to our immune systems.

What a sad state of affairs for a country with such wealth and abundance. This state of affairs and my deep desire to see every person be the whole person God created them to be has led me to write this book. It is only a small beginning. Much, much more could and must be written to teach Americans how to restore and build the health of our future — our children.

Not one parent that I know would consciously choose to poison or kill his/her child. Yet, out of ignorance, misinformation and stressful schedules, more parents than not are doing just that.

A child's food choices are established by the eating habits found at home. You impact the future of your child and the inheritance you leave them by what you feed them. The most valuable inheritance you can give them is a life of health to live out their full and complete destiny. A sick and diseased child has little, if any, bright future to look forward to.

Is this too dramatic? Take time to really look at your baby, child, teen, or spouse. Are they really healthy, sparkling, and alert? Do they have shiny eyes, good clear complexions, appropriate weight, and peaceful, calm countenances? Are they a delight to be around (most of the time)? If not, this book has some valuable information for you and your child.

Is it possible to raise a healthy child without being Betty Crocker? Is it possible to enjoy health without spending all day in the kitchen or all of your household budget on food? It is possible, because our family has done it, as well as many other families. It is possible for you to do it, too!

We started when we were unemployed and living on a total income of less than $850.00 a month. I was dying from depression, weight problems and a host of mental, emotional, and physical ailments. The tools I give you in *Kid Smart!* helped us and have helped a host of other families make a dramatic difference in the health of their children and themselves.

It is possible... so let's begin!

A Letter to Your Child from Anna

Dear Friends,

Hi! My name is Anna Townsley. I am 10 years old. I'm here to tell you about health food. To you health food may sound strange, but it's not. My mom, Cheryl Townsley, almost died because of what she ate. I would not have a mom unless she had started to eat healthy. That's why I choose to eat healthy. I don't ever want to go through what she did.

Health food is not just low in fat. It's not sugar, aspartame, white bread, or yellow cheese. It's not junk food. It is lots of fruits and vegetables. It is lots of water and juices without sugar.

There are lots of reasons you should eat healthy. Here are three reasons:

1. Healthy food keeps you strong and healthy.
2. You live longer.
3. You don't get as sick.

There are lots of reasons why I eat healthy. I have already told you three reasons, and here are three more:

1. Because my parents eat healthy.
2. Because it's good for my body.
3. Because after 10 years, I've never been to the doctor for being sick.

Are you still wanting to know why you should eat health food? Here's three more reasons:

1. You have more energy.
2. For some of you, it makes your parents happy.
3. It makes your brain work better.

Your friend,

Anna Townsley

—☆—

A Letter to Dad From Forest

Health is a family adventure — not a family battle! As with all adventures, someone has to be the leader — someone has to set the direction. Effective leadership will make any adventure a success, regardless of the trials encountered. Unfortunately, what all too often happens is strife and conflict set in and your adventure turns into a disaster. Is this the case in your home? Are your adventures, your dreams, turning into nightmares?

As we work with families who are struggling in the area of health, the core problem is almost always a lack of leadership, direction, and vision. Instead of bringing unity and joy to a family, the issue of health usually brings discord — one spouse gets excited, the other gets resistant and then, POW! All too often dads are the source of this strife (if this doesn't apply to you, please don't be offended — be thankful)!

So dads, let's look at what we can do. What is our role? During the first 10 years of our marriage the role I resisted the most was being the husband — providing the leadership and direction that my family so desperately needed. The result was on going confusion and conflict. Please listen carefully, I am not at all suggesting or encouraging men to move into the stereotypical role of dictatorial leadership. This is the role that has created so many problems in our society. Being a leader implies that someone is following you — out of a heart desire, not because, "I have to because I fear you!"

As a leader your job is to bring your family into unity and focused purpose. A family operating in unity is truly an unstoppable force. It is a joy to be a part of a united family. What you can accomplish as such a team is truly unlimited. Somehow we seem to be able to do this at work or even in sports, but not at home. Today it is time to turn your attention toward home — with a bit of effort and commitment you can dramatically turn around your family's health.

Cheryl's books, *Food Smart!* and *Kid Smart!* will give you the tools you need. It is possible to have a healthy, happy, united family, but it requires effort. You may need to learn to do things you've never done before, but I can assure you, it's worth it! I've been on both sides of the fence and I wouldn't trade where I'm at now for anything.

May the Lord bless you with a vision of health and prosperity for you and your family!

A Dad who cares,

Forest Townsley

—☆—

Part One:

Changing More Than Diapers!

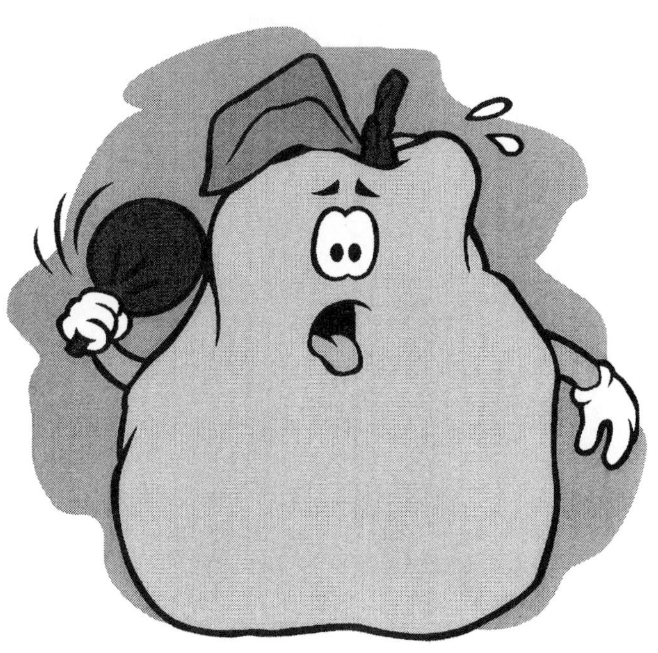

CHAPTER ONE

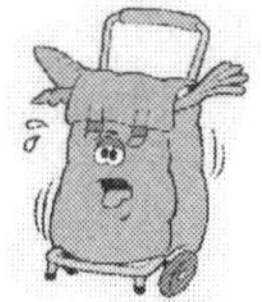

Anything worth doing contains a seed of greatness bound by a hard shell. When that hard shell is shattered, unstoppable life pours forth.

Go Beyond the "I Can't" to the "I Can!"

When I meet with parents and adults throughout the country, I often hear objections as to why health can't work for their "unique" situation. The first step in getting you and your family healthy is to identify the objections in your life and tackle them one by one. If you leave them uncovered, they will rise up and sabotage your best efforts to change. Do not leave this chapter without knowing why you have ignored health in the past.

One of the most misunderstood aspects of successfully changing an area in your life is the realization that change is a process. Change does not occur by pushing the button of a microlife. Nor does it occur by rubbing on a magical cream or by popping some power-punched pill. Change requires effort, time, and commitment.

When I look back over the years since 1990, since my total collapse, I am amazed at the progress we've made. I reached the bottom of my pit in 1989. My fast-paced lifestyle, poor eating habits, difficult pregnancy and stress had culminated in a collapse of my physical, mental, emotional, and financial well-being. In the few short years prior to 1989, we went through bankruptcy, foreclosure on our house, unemployment, and my suicide attempt.

At that point I was a little short on hope that any change would work in my life, especially as a woman and a mom. I felt totally inadequate to be dear little Anna's mother. She was (and is) so precious. What a wonderful bundle of blessing from the Lord she was. But, what was she doing in my life? Answers seemed far away.

With my life such a mess, how could I possibly pass on anything of value to a daughter? How could I even know what to do? Was there an answer? *Yes!* A step at a time, we were introduced to the principles that restored my health. *Food Smart!* gives you my story as an individual and my fight to regain my health.

In *Kid Smart!* I'm here to help you learn about health as a parent. When you first hold that little bundle of red, wrinkled skin with the loud cry, many emotions can flood your soul. From ecstasy to delight to fear to disinterest, a myriad of emotions clamor for your attention.

I was no different. I was so tired from an extended (to put it mildly) labor that I verged on the edge of disinterest. Forest, on the other hand, was commanding the nurses how to handle "his" perfect little girl. They obviously had no idea how to do it "right" the Townsley way.

At that point, we had only begun to see my downward health spiral. I had yet to completely fall apart or attempt suicide. So, our road to health had many stumbling blocks ahead. Yet, if I could forge ahead, find the way and overcome those obstacles, so can you. My objections were as plentiful, if not more so, than yours. If I could overcome mine, I know you can overcome yours!

Take the time to begin to identify your objections to change and/or health. That may seem simplistic and even unnecessary. Yet, our family has learned over and over again that if we are serious about a change, we must take the time to explore and identify our areas of resistance. If we do not identify the resistance, name it and replace it, then it will ambush us at our weakest moment.

Once you begin to identify your areas of resistance (and even that is an on-going process), write it down. A great prophet, Habakkuk, said, "Write the vision plainly, for all to see." Writing on paper your areas of resistance and your plans to change removes some of the power of the problem and transfers that power to the solution. It also helps clarify what it is that keeps you from successfully changing. This is especially important as a parent.

As a parent, we become quite busy with the daily activities of parenting. The thought of adding another "job," like eating healthy, seem impossible to fit into our day. When I first became a parent, I was amazed at how full 24 hours became. Motherhood was far more taxing than any corporate position I had ever held. Changing in the area of health, especially as a busy mom, represented some of the most difficult change I have ever experienced.

So, don't feel isolated if the changes in *Kid Smart!* at first seem a little bit much. Remember, we spent four years making a mess and the next six years cleaning up that mess. And we still have wonderful opportunities to grow. (I smile and groan when I say that!)

Give yourself permission to take time to know where you are, what you don't like, and what you want to change in the area of health. Take time to learn to look at your life with new eyes. Learn to hear what you are saying about your life, your child, and health.

LET'S LOOK AT SOME COMMON OBJECTIONS

When someone suggests "health and nutrition for children," do you find yourself running for cover? Does the word *health* conjure up a picture of a "fruit-and-granola-strange-type" person in your mind's eye? Maybe you hear yourself saying, I can't get our family healthy because:

- "My schedule is too busy!"
- "My kids are picky eaters."
- "Nutrition is too confusing."
- "Health food is too expensive."
- "It's too hard."

Have you heard yourself utter these statements? They are not the real stumbling block, they only represent the first level of excuses. They are the old mind-sets that keep you from moving forward into health.

They are real, but they aren't the core issue. What do I mean? Each of these statements really represents the fact that health has a lower priority than how you currently spend your time and money. Let's take each of these statements, individually, and look at the mind-set and value system that it really represents. Let's explode the surface objection, so you can move with some freedom into the real core issues. As you resolve the core issues, you will move both you and your child into health.

"My Schedule is Too Busy!"

This statement says that a schedule cannot be changed and is more important than the health of your child. We would never come right out and say that. However, that is the core belief behind the words. We resist changing our schedule because we do not believe in or value the possible result. Or, the apparent price seems too high.

A NEW WAY OF THINKING

Time is the one asset we each have the exact, finite amount of, whether we are sick or healthy. How we spend our time is what varies from person to person. Sick people spend time differently than healthy people. This is true at the point of sickness, it is also true of the time prior to any sickness. Likewise, it is quite true of parents of sick and parents of healthy children.

It takes a great deal of time to stay home with a sick child. It takes time to plan, prepare, and serve healthy food. One is a price, one is an investment. One approach drains you, one provides an on-going return.

Health gives us more time to do what we want to do. When health replaces sickness, you will be amazed at how much more time you have. If you are dealing with chronic sickness, doctor's visits, and stress, you must take a look at your schedule. Something has to give — either what you are doing or *you.* *Food Smart!* spends a whole chapter helping you learn how to simplify your life and find pockets of time for change to occur.

"My Kids are Picky Eaters."

Who taught them to eat that way? If you allowed them to be picky, you are probably a picky eater yourself. Or, you don't really care enough about what your child eats to require any other behavior.

If we demand well-balanced eating of ourselves, yet allow our children to eat whatever they want, we are allowing a double standard. If we demand well-balanced eating of our children, but not of ourselves, we are, again, allowing a double standard. This dual standard will lead to confusion and instability. "A double-minded person is unstable in all of his ways."

A NEW WAY OF THINKING

Children will always eat food that is either appealing or eaten by the rest of the family with obvious enjoyment. Chapters 4 and 5 will give you many tips and strategies on how to make food appealing to any age group. The recipes chapters will give you many actual recipes guaranteed to taste so good you won't have to fake your pleasure.

Some children are picky because they don't feel good when they eat. This is often a sign of allergies instead of just rebellion. Take your child to a health care provider who will examine your child for allergies. Removing those allergenic foods could cause such relief that the child's appetite blossoms.

Other children use food as a means of control. They refuse to eat some food(s) knowing that, given time, you will always cave in. The issue here is not food, it is consistent parenting. Make a decision as to the approach you want to use. Then, stick with it and be consistent. Children will push limits to see how serious you are. You are the decision maker as the parent, not the child. That means you have the responsibility as to the outcome of your decision.

"Nutrition is Too Confusing."

Yes, there is a great deal of information on health and nutrition in today's world. However, the basic principles are quite simple. Mathematics start with the basics of addition and subtraction. You can move into great complexity by the time you get into calculus, but the basics have never changed. *Kid Smart!* will give you the basics. Then, you can decide how advanced you want to become on the subject of health. The basics allow you to get started and make significant progress.

A NEW WAY OF THINKING

Chapter 6 will explain nutrition with simple addition and subtraction methods — what to add and what to remove from your diet. Chapter 7 will help you apply this to different age groups (a little multiplication and division). Chapter 11 will help you know what to substitute for your child's favorite foods.

Start right where you are and make healthier choices, one step at a time. You don't need a degree in nutrition. Nor do you need to implement every possible step in one fell swoop (which is impossible anyway).

The basics are the key. You need to know the basics of what to add and remove from you and your child's current lifestyle. Start right where you are. Don't accept the lie that you have to understand every aspect of nutrition to start. If you had followed that philosophy, you would never have gone to first grade without knowing calculus.

"Health Food is Too Expensive."

Ask the question, "Expensive compared to what?" Sickness and premature death cost great pain and millions of dollars in America today. Being home from work to care for a sick child costs time and money. Doctor bills and prescriptions cost money.

Meat, dairy, sodas, and high fat snack items are some of the most expensive foods in a grocery store. Health food — too expensive — compared to what?

A NEW WAY OF THINKING

When I mentally, physically, and emotionally collapsed, the cost to my family was extensive. It cost Forest time and money to care for the house and for me. It cost our daughter the sense of security, hope, and comfort a healthy mother is designed to provide. It nearly cost me my life. Sickness is very expensive!

When we made the decision to pursue health, we were on a limited budget (less than $850/month). We were on a limited time budget (I was sick and had minimal energy). If we can come through those financial barriers, so can you.

The issue is not that health food is too expensive. The real issue is how do you want to spend your money. If you make a decision to eat healthy food, your creativity will come to your rescue. The recipes in this book and my other cookbooks are designed to work on right budgets. We also have several meal planning products available through our Lifestyle for Health office. Call us at 303-771-9357 for more details.

"It's Too Hard."

Many of us believe that if something is too hard we aren't "called" to do it. Is living with sickness and the threat of cancer easy? How do you respond to your children's excuse that a school assignment is "too hard?" In our home, that excuse doesn't go very far.

How does your boss respond to your complaint that a job is "too hard?" What happens if you are your own boss and find a job "too hard?" As a manager, how do you respond to an employee who says a job is "too hard?" Being "too hard" is a relative statement.

A NEW WAY OF THINKING

What a lie to think that we can't do something because it is "too hard." Stop fussing and start *thinking*. We applaud the person who walks away from welfare to become a successful entrepreneur. We applaud the gold medal Olympic champion who stands on his/her podium of success. Why? Fulfilled potential in others strikes a cord of desire in our heart of hearts.

What if babies decided walking was "too hard?" Would they have ever taken that first step and fallen down? Do we focus on their first steps or their subsequent falls? We are ecstatic with their steps. We applaud their success with all of our might. These precious children have just demonstrated a powerful truth — anything worth doing contains a seed of greatness bound by a hard shell. When that shell is shattered through effort, unstoppable life pours forth. Don't let the shell of "too hard" keep you from the life that is inside that shell. Crack that shell with determination. You and your child will never be the same — life will pour forth as you have never known it before.

LET'S START WITH YOU!

Someone paid for this book. You are reading it. If you don't take the time here and now to address your areas of resistance, reading the rest of the book will be a waste of your irreplaceable time. Why? You will read each word through the filter of the shell of your excuses. Expose those excuses and you will begin to see the potential contained within. The potential that a creative God placed in you at your birth and within your child at his/her birth.

If you choose to identify and address your excuses you will learn much from this book. The number of issues or objections that you have is not the size of your mountain. The strength of your desire to change is the size of your opportunity. So open up to "a new way of thinking."

LET'S DEFINE A FEW WORDS

To help you pursue health, it is important to make sure that we are using the same words. Let's define a few key terms so that we can communicate more accurately.

Health (for a child or adult) includes:
energy for all activities and a surplus for recreation, good appetite and digestion, healthy eyes, shiny skin and shiny hair, a healthy colon with regular bowel movements, good memory and clear thinking, freedom from worry and anxiety, the ability to relax and enjoy what you are doing, freedom from dis-ease, spontaneous humor and laughter

Sickness (for a child or adult) includes:
not feeling good, requiring regular medication (including non-

prescription drugs), a sense of constant tiredness, weight problems (whether overweight or underweight), looking less than your best on a regular basis, mood swings and regular irritability, constant stress, rigid emotions, body odor, indigestion and bloating, and the list goes on and on and on....

Nutrition includes:
cleansing or cleaning the body of toxins and poisons. *Food Smart!* has an entire section dedicated to cleansing. We have cleansing products available through our Lifestyle for Health office. Call us at 303-771-9357 for details.

Building is:
providing the necessary building blocks for strong bones, teeth, cells, organs, and bodily systems. This can include nutrients found in wholesome food, pure water, rest, exercise, and supplements. We will address each of these building blocks throughout *Kid Smart!*

What has kept you from improving the health of you or your children? What is the seemingly impossible barrier in your life? Do you want that barrier shattered and forever removed?

Take the time to do the following exercise to help build your health opportunity. Write your responses on paper. That may seem unnecessary, but it does yield significant results. Once an enemy is defined and a plan of defense mounted — with complete commitment to see it through with God's help — you are guaranteed success. The only variable is when the success will manifest.

Identifying your fears, excuses, and stumbling blocks is defining the enemy. It's giving it a name. It gives the problem definition. In math, once the problem is defined (correctly), given the right help, it can be solved.

Kid Smart! helps you with the plan of action. You must define the problem. God wants you to be a winner. You have a very precious creation in your life… your child. Let's combine our desire to change with His power to help us change. With such a winning combination, we are sure to bring a destiny of life and health to our children.

QUESTIONS FOR YOU TO THINK ABOUT AND RESPOND TO

1. What holds you back from pursuing health?
2. What is the biggest obstacle or fear you face in changing what you or your family eats?
3. Why does it seem so impossible?

MOTIVATORS TO HELP YOU CHANGE YOUR MIND-SET

Some of these motivators were introduced to us by Peter J. Daniels in his book *How To Be Motivated All The Time*. I have added to them to make them apply to you and to health.

- Know that others have successfully brought health into their lives (the Townsleys). Therefore, it is possible for you to do it, too.
- Decide to act motivated about health, and your emotions will begin to follow.
- Replace negative self-talk (I can't do it because…) with positive statements of encouragement. You decide what you say and what you think about… no one else does.
- Realize that as you build the health of your child, you are giving him/her an inheritance that money can't buy.
- You and your children have a purpose to be alive and healthy.
- No one can stop you or your children from getting healthier, if you really want to be healthier. God's grace

is sufficient to carry you through, if you are in agreement and participating in the change process.

KEY APPLICATION

- ••• Look at each of your responses to the first three questions.
- ••• Reread the motivators.
- ••• Now, how else could you respond to these three questions?

As you honestly look at your areas of resistance, begin to identify a new way of living. As you learn that you were created to be more than an overcomer, you will be introduced to the Author of Life.

The resistance you have had in the past is the hard shell that has kept you from experiencing success. As that hard shell melts away in the face of the vision of who you were created to be, you are shattering that hard shell. Watch out! New life will begin to multiply and transform you.

Now let that new life pour forth from that shattered old shell. Open up to being a new creation… you and your child.

CHAPTER TWO

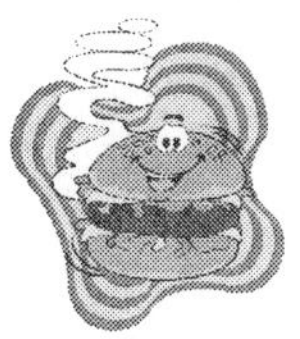

Today's parents are ignoring the blinking yellow lights of sickness and disease in our children's generation.

Kids... Health Food... Why Bother?

"It has long been recognized that the eating patterns and the foods to which children are exposed in the early years of life are among the most influential factors determining their nutritional health as adults." — The Child Nutritional Advisory Council

Parents determine the health of their children from as early as the time of conception. The health of the parents at the time the child is conceived critically impacts the health of the fetus and the newborn baby. From as early as birth, children eat the food their parents give them, whether it is breast milk or formula. Children learn to adopt the eating patterns of their parents. During the formative years of infant, toddler, and school age, children are dependent upon their parent(s) for their food, housing, and emotional support.

Is the attitude, knowledge, and action of a parent important to the health of a child? Obviously, yes! Yet, today many American parents are ignoring the blinking yellow lights of sickness and disease in our children's generation. What is the over-all health picture of today's average child? It's not as rosy as we'd like to believe.

- ••• 1 in 6 children are seriously deficient in calcium. (needed for strong bones and teeth)
- ••• 1 in 3 children are deficient in iron. (needed for energy, immune system, attention span)
- ••• Nearly 1 in 2 children are deficient in zinc. (needed for immune function, skin, healthy sexual development, wound healing, overall growth, and blood pressure regulation)
- ••• Over 9 in 10 children are lacking magnesium. (needed for bone and muscle formation, nervous system, and blood pressure regulation)
- ••• 1 in 6 children lack vitamin A. (needed for tissue repair and maintenance, and immune system)
- ••• Nearly 1 in 2 children are seriously deficient in vitamin C. (needed for skin, digestion, healing, vitamin and mineral metabolism.)
- ••• 1 in 7 children lack vitamin B-12. (needed for nervous system, formation of RNA and DNA, and metabolism)
- ••• 1 in 5 children lack folic acid. (needed for blood cell formation, collagen building, and metabolism)
- ••• Nearly 3 million children between the ages of 6 and 17 years suffer from high blood pressure.

— summarized from the *Vitamin Supplement Journal*

Beyond these deficiencies, 60% of American children are overweight. According to the American Heart Association, even with our newest low-fat obsession, obesity has increased by 54% in children aged 6 to 11 and 39% in ages 12 to 17.

At the other end of the spectrum are the children with eating disorders. Starving and bingeing tendencies are now hitting at younger and younger ages. The low-fat obsession in this country has caused us to compare ourselves to anorexic media models. These bone-thin models have become our definition of health and our picture of the ideal body weight.

Weight, whether over or under, is nearly always a symptom of being out of balance. When the health issue is identified and treated, weight will usually take care of itself. Focusing on weight, without addressing the health root, will rarely cause weight to balance and (the key) maintain itself.

I was appalled to learn that 24% of the children studied by the National Cancer Institute ate no fruit the previous day and 25% had eaten no vegetables. Fruits and vegetables are the basis for much of our needed nutrition, yet 24 – 25% of our children have no fruits and vegetables on a single day.

In today's culture, most of what children learn about anything, including nutrition, is from television. The media, along with schools and peers, has left our children subject to myths, lies, and confusion. It is time for parents to understand enough about health and nutrition that they can be an example and a role model to their children. Often, parents are as uneducated or as misinformed as their children when it comes to the subject of health.

The National Cancer Institute's research indicates that children between grades 2 and 6 have the following beliefs about nutrition:

- 15% believe cheese is a good source of fiber (it isn't).
- 48% believe apple juice has more fat than whole milk (it doesn't).

- 36% believe watermelon has more fat than American cheese (it doesn't).

Where does this leave us? It leaves us with uneducated children who are becoming slaves to a poor quality of health, if not total sickness and disease. What is the alternative?

There are some children who do not fit those statistics and will die prematurely. Our daughter, along with many other children, has not seen a doctor for years (except to have her chin sewn from a fall), has never had an ear infection, has never taken an antibiotic, and is bright and alert. These children are a growing group of youngsters who have parents who are taking an active role in their children's health. It is possible and it is important. As the adult in your child's life, regardless of the child's age, you have the responsibility and opportunity to tremendously impact the health of that child.

The following self-test can help you to examine your overall health and the health of your child. Take the time to examine each person in your family in light of these symptoms. Remember, symptoms are not just an annoying intrusion to erase and suppress. They are your body's way of communicating that you have a problem. Ignoring symptoms guarantees you will have to deal with a crisis... the question is merely *when* the crisis will come.

SELF -TEST: HOW HEALTHY ARE YOU?

Rate each of the following symptoms as to how often you or your child experience it.

Point Scale:

0 = Never or almost never experience the symptom
1 = Occasionally experience the symptom
2 = Frequently experience the symptom

HEAD

- ❑ headaches
- ❑ faintness
- ❑ dizziness
- ❑ insomnia

subtotal ____

MIND

- ❑ poor memory
- ❑ confusion
- ❑ poor concentration
- ❑ poor coordination
- ❑ difficulty making decisions
- ❑ stuttering, stammering
- ❑ slurred speech
- ❑ learning disabilities

subtotal ____

EYES

- ❑ watery, itchy eyes
- ❑ swollen, reddened, or sticky eyelids
- ❑ dark circles under eyes
- ❑ blurred vision
- ❑ continually deteriorating vision

subtotal ____

EARS

- ❑ itchy ears
- ❑ earaches or ear infections
- ❑ ear drainage
- ❑ ringing in the ears
- ❑ hearing loss

subtotal ____

NOSE/MOUTH

- ❑ stuffy nose
- ❑ sinus problems
- ❑ gagging or frequent need to clear throat
- ❑ sore throat, hoarseness
- ❑ swollen, white, or discolored tongue, gums, or lips
- ❑ canker sores

subtotal ____

LUNGS

- ❑ congestion
- ❑ asthma, bronchitis
- ❑ shortness of breath
- ❑ difficulty in breathing

subtotal ____

HEART

- ❑ skipped heartbeat
- ❑ rapid heartbeats
- ❑ high blood pressure

subtotal ____

JOINTS /MUSCLES

- ❑ aching or painful joints
- ❑ arthritis
- ❑ stiff, limited movement
- ❑ feeling weak or tired

subtotal ____

SKIN

- ❑ acne
- ❑ hives, rashes, dry spots on skin
- ❑ hair loss
- ❑ flushing or hot flashes
- ❑ excessive sweating

❑ lack of sweating

subtotal ____

DIGESTION

❑ nausea or vomiting
❑ diarrhea
❑ constipation
❑ bloated feeling
❑ belching, passing of gas
❑ heartburn

subtotal ____

ENERGY/ACTIVITY

❑ fatigue
❑ hyperactive
❑ restless

subtotal ____

EMOTIONS

❑ mood swings
❑ anxiety, fear, nervousness
❑ irritable, fearful, insecure
❑ depression

subtotal ____

WEIGHT

❑ binge eating or drinking
❑ food cravings
❑ excessive weight
❑ under weight
❑ compulsive eating
❑ water retention

subtotal ____

OTHER

❑ frequent illness

- ❑ frequent urination
- ❑ genital itch or discharge
- ❑ red cheeks
- ❑ dull skin and eyes

subtotal ____
TOTAL ____

If any individual section subtotals are more than 5 or the total is more than 25, you or your child has health problems that need to be addressed. Your choice is whether you will deal with them now in more of a preventative mode or later as a health care crisis.

Kids... health food... why bother? Wholesome food, pure water, quality supplementation, and lifestyle habits are the keys that can keep you and your child from being one of the statistics found at the beginning of this chapter.

QUESTIONS FOR YOU TO THINK ABOUT AND RESPOND TO

1. What was my score on the above test? What was the score of each member of my family?
2. Given that score and the statistics in this chapter how do I honestly perceive my health and the health of my family?
3. Is that health picture significant to me?

MOTIVATORS TO HELP YOU CHANGE

- ••• You are the key to making a health change in your family.
- ••• Your health today reflects your health investment yesterday.
- ••• What you invest in your health today determines the rest of your life.

••• A healthy future comes from paying the price of discipline today.

KEY APPLICATIONS

••• Look at each of your responses to the above three questions.

••• Reread the motivators.

••• Are you willing to commit time and dollars to change your current health picture? Quantify the time and dollars you are willing to spend.

••• Determine the value (in dollars and significance) of producing a healthy child, able to face the future and live out a destiny.

••• You have just written the will and inheritance you are willing to pass on to your child. Just as you would with any will, have it notarized by someone else. Include some other person (i.e., the father, mother, grandparent, etc.) in this will for your child.

CHAPTER THREE

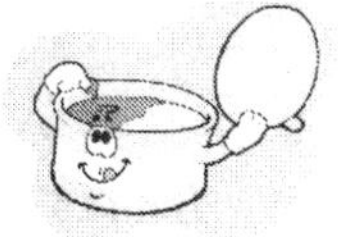

If you give yourself permission to take time to learn a new way of living, you can avoid the guilt of not being perfect.

Where Do I Start?

According to the 1988 Surgeon General's Report on nutrition and health: 68% of all deaths in the U.S. each year are due to nutrition-related diseases!

Getting healthy requires a look at what we eat, when we eat, how we eat, and our overall emotional, spiritual, and mental environment. We are what we assimilate (digest and absorb). We are each also a spirit with a soul (mind, will, and emotions) in a body. All three must function in order to be a whole person operating in health.

Getting healthy is a process, not a destination. As I share the steps that will help get you, your child, and your family healthy, remember, you can only do it "one step at a time." Trying to do everything all at once starting today will only result in confusion, frustration, and paralysis. So, don't bother to try and do everything at once. Pick the step that works best for you right where you are. One step will lead to the next step. One step at a time, you are moving in the *direction* of health.

Since health is a process, give yourself permission to take time to learn how to become healthier and to develop health in your children. If you decide to give yourself permission to take time to learn a new way of living, you can avoid the guilt of not being perfect the first day. If you are in a life-threatening crisis such as I was, get help immediately. Time is now your most vital commodity.

The following steps are in the order that I have found yields the best results. Do not overlook the importance of the first several steps. Implementation strategies, by age group, are given in the next chapter.

STEP 1: MAKE A DECISION TO PURSUE HEALTH.

We are free-will creatures with the freedom of choice. A decision is when you exercise that freedom and determine the direction you are taking in a given area. Without a decision you will waffle between "I should" and "I can't."

A decision is when you make up your mind and the issue is settled. You have the right to chose what you eat, drink, believe and think about. If you have not made a decision, then each meal or opportunity to eat requires a new decision with unlimited choices. This takes more energy, time, and effort. A decision limits choices to only those that will support your decision.

Make a decision. You can choose life or death. The right to choose is yours. Healthy people make the decision to pursue health. That decision sets their direction and begins to define their course.

STEP 2: GET IN UNITY!

Many times I have watched a parent (mother or father) see the purpose in getting their family healthy. Their eyes take on the gleam of a zealot. They announce their decision to their unsuspecting family. *Wham!* Instant rebellion and mutiny in the house. What happened?

Health is a personal issue from toddlerhood to adulthood and every step in between. You cannot announce to a family that "they *are* going to get healthy." This is a direction that requires a team commitment.

If a family is to successfully pursue health, both parents must be in agreement. If the mom is excited and dad isn't, I can guarantee you the kids will eat what dad eats. Mom will be left preparing two meals — what a time waster. If dad is excited and mom isn't, sabotage will occur at every meal. A lack of unity at this point makes moving to the next step a waste of time and energy.

What can you do? Sit down and talk about why you want to get healthier and why you want the children to get healthier. Communication is key to bring about unity. You may have to go slower than you would like. Unity at a slower pace is far wiser than rebellion at the speed of light.

Taking the time to get in unity at this point will save hours of tears, frustrations, and problems later. Unity requires that all the people involved have made the same decision, from their hearts. A home divided — falls. A home united — stands.

STEP 3: INCLUDE YOUR CHILDREN.

If you are starting this process while you are pregnant or with infants, you are blessed and fortunate. You can build health into your child right from the start. What a tremendous head start and blessing!

However, if you are starting with a toddler, school-age child, teen, or "bigger child," you have a different opportunity. It is important that your children buy into this health process or you will continually be in a battle of wills.

Since every family operates differently in their parenting, how you involve your children will vary. The implementation strategies in the next chapter will give you many ideas as to how to introduce health at different ages. It is key to remember that children copy their parents. If you have truly made a decision and are excited, eventually, if included, your children will catch your enthusiasm.

The key here is to not overlook the importance of even a toddler wanting to participate in this process. When our nine-year-old daughter went through a period of rebellion over health food, we had to stop and reevaluate how to include her in the health process.

What did we do? We got her involved. We developed a plan and got some outside help, with her involvement every step of the way. Today, only a few months later, we are seeing victories in her choices far beyond where we were when we "made" her eat healthy. She now owns her decision and she is excited about the results she is getting with her decision.

Get creative. If you know that prayer works, pray. Ask the Lord to give you creative ideas to involve your child in getting healthy. You will be amazed at the simple ideas that will begin to bubble up.

STEP 4: EXAMINE YOUR FOOD TRADITIONS.

When you begin the process of getting healthy, many insignificant-appearing events stand ready to defeat you. What about holidays? Birthday cake? Parties? What about the old stand by of 7-Up and a cracker for an upset stomach? So many traditions and habits will stand quietly on the side lines waiting to come in and knock you down.

Take the time to list the many activities your family does that include food. As you learn how to make healthier substitutions (later in this chapter), determine which activities you will work on. Develop a plan to handle each potential saboteur. If you don't, you will be caught off guard; your child will suffer.

When Anna attends the Harvest Festival at our church, she is prepared. We have talked about the sugar-based candy that will be there. She gets to select her favorite alternatives at our health food store. We talk to her about the choices that will be available to her. We discuss the consequences she will face if she dumps a bunch of candy into her body. A body that hasn't had that kind of candy will get sick and she is the one who will get sick, not me. As a result of this process, she is developing character that far exceeds many adults.

Have a family-agreed-upon plan for holidays, vacations, grandparent visits, parties, and other potential problem areas. Encourage your children to be creative in your family solutions. The plans do not have to start perfect. The key is to continually be moving toward better health.

STEP 5: IDENTIFY THE COST OF CHANGE.

Unfortunately many people will never change unless they are miserable enough. Many parents do not look at helping their children get healthier until they are involved in a health crisis. Are you one of those people?

If you are wanting to make a change, count the cost of staying where you are. How much money is spent in doctor visits and medication? How much time do you spend "doctoring" a child who is home sick? How many family fights originate from unstable emotions induced by food allergies and sensitivities? What is the emotional cost to you in raising a "hyper" child? What is the emotional cost to you and your overweight child in dealing with cruel comments by other children? The list goes on and on. Count the cost.

If the cost is significant to you, it will help motivate you to make a change. If you see no cost in your current situation, you have a minimal chance of successfully making any change.

Another way to count the cost to determine what you are missing out on by not being healthy. Is your child missing out on academic success because of continual fatigue and sickness? Will your child miss out on becoming an adult because of cancer? Will your child potentially face prison because of uncontrollable emotions triggered by food sensitivities and excess medication?

Count the cost both in money and lost opportunities. Don't let that loss be vague and easily overlooked. Take a hard look at what you as a parent are causing your child to live without. Do not move into guilt, move into action to know you can make a difference in his/her life!

STEP 6: ESTABLISH THE PRICE YOU ARE WILLING TO PAY.

You have made a decision. You know the cost of staying where you are. Now you must establish the price you are willing to pay to change. That price includes money, time, and the pain of change.

By now you know that no "June Cleaver" in shining apron is going to appear in your home to handle all your health issues. Changing what you eat, how you pursue health and fight sickness requires a commitment to handle the pain of change.

I can help identify the steps and the necessary action to become healthier. You must pay the price on a daily basis to implement those steps. That is akin to exercise. Learning to say yes to wise food choices and no to poor food choices is an exercise in self discovery and discipline. I would be lying if I said that that process is without any pain.

As a woman and mother, I know the pain of childbirth. It was painful. However, the result of that pain is a beautiful girl with life and future generations to follow. Did I enjoy the pain? Of course not! Do I enjoy the fruit of that pain? You bet I do. She is a joy and a blessing.

Are you willing to pay the price in time, money, and pain to help your child have life? Only you can determine what price you are willing and able to pay.

STEP 7: DEVELOP AN ATTITUDE.

As parents we know that attitude is everything. Attitude development in a home starts with the parents. Your attitude (and your child's) will either propel you forward or drag you back. Your attitude is your mind-set that says who you really are.

A positive attitude committed to health helps you seek solutions rather than bag out with excuses. Your attitude represents your glasses that help you focus on either the problem or the solution. Your attitude will multiply in your child.

If you think you can command health while your attitude on health is marginal, forget it. Children have a way of knowing what you really believe. At least be honest enough to tell your children where you really are. This may not be where you want to be, but only through honesty and family commitment can all of you successfully move to a new attitude.

STEP 8: BEGIN TO ADD.

Remember the rule that math is based on the basics of addition and subtraction? Well health is also based on addition and subtraction. In my book *Food Smart!* I go into much more detail on what to add and why. However, here I want to help you know which foods to add in what sequence in your pursuit of health. The next chapter will deal with food additions by age.

First of all, it is critical to *add more fruits and vegetables* to your family's diet. Fruits are cleansing and a key source of vitamins. Vegetables help build the body and are a key source of vitamins and minerals. When fruits and vegetables are *eaten raw* or in fresh juice, they provide a rich supply of enzymes. Enzymes are the "spark plugs" to make your body run and unlock the energy contained in minerals and vitamins. Heat, in the form of cooking or processing, kills most enzymes.

Secondly, *organic produce* is the best for children. Children, due to their smaller body size, are much more vulnerable to the pesticides and chemicals found on produce. Many nutritionists claim that organic produce contains two to nine times the nutrition of produce grown on nutrient-deficient land. If organic produce is not available to you, try to get locally grown (fresh, with less shipping time) produce. You can also wash your produce to help remove the oil-based pesticides. (I use a few drops of Shaklee Basic H in a sink full of water. Soak the produce for 10 to 20 minutes. Rinse, drain, and dry. Bag the produce and store in the refrigerator. The produce will last much longer, taste fresher, and have fewer chemicals.)

Third, *add more whole grains, beans, raw nuts, seeds, and sprouts to your food intake.* Whole grains are especially rich in the B vitamin complex, which helps the nerves. Beans are an excellent source of protein. Seeds help feed the brain and the reproductive system. Be careful of nut butters (peanut butter is highest in fat and usually contains sugar). Almond butter is a much better choice. Sprouts are the most "live" food available. My books *Food Smart!* and the *Lifestyle for Health* cookbook address these foods in much more detail.

Fourth, *add more pure water*. Many people unknowingly have health problems directly linked to dehydration. Sodas actually act as a diuretic. A child who only drinks sodas, sweetened juice, and milk is probably deficient in healthy fluids.

Water is key for mental functioning, cellular activities, and many other bodily functions.

To determine an approximate amount of water intake for your child:

- Your child's weight divided by 2 = # of ounces to consume daily.
- This total divided by 8 = total # of glasses to drink each day.

As much as possible avoid tap water and use either distilled or reverse osmosis (RO) water. A home filter system can be purchased or you can purchase bottled, distilled, or RO water from grocery stores.

Fifth, depending on the age and current health status of your child, *supplementation* may need to be added. Any supplement should be natural and not synthetic. Be sure you know the quality of the product and the integrity of the manufacturer. I would not recommend chewable vitamins from grocery stores. They are usually loaded with sugar, colorings, chemicals, and synthetic ingredients. My book *Meals in 30 Minutes* discusses our family approach to supplementation.

STEP 9: BEGIN TO SUBTRACT.

There are numerous items that can come out of your life that will make a noticeable difference in your child's health and behavior. I will present several so that you can work on the ones that best match your family and then move on to the others. Remember, one step in the right direction is much better than becoming paralyzed trying to do everything.

First, *eliminate or minimize foods processed with chemicals.* This includes preservatives, food coloring, MSG, and nitrates. In order to know if food has these chemicals, check the label.

Food coloring usually is quickly recognized by the use of a number. MSG can be shown as MSG or one of its aliases (Accent, Vetsin, Chinese seasoning, Flutavene, RL-50, hydrolyzed vegetable protein (HVP), hydrolyzed plant protein, natural flavors (may be HVP), or flavorings). These ingredients are not recognized, digested, or assimilated by the body. They become toxic and are stored in fat tissue.

Second, *eliminate or minimize hydrogenated fat products.* This includes margarine (butter is easier for the body to digest), shortenings, and all products using hydrogenated or partially hydrogenated fats (these will be shown on the labels). Hydrogenated oils or fats have had a molecule of hydrogen added. This makes the product close to plastic, which the body cannot handle.

The alternative to hydrogenated fats and oil is expeller pressed oils. These oils have not had hydrogen or petroleum solvents added to them. If a product is expeller pressed, it will say so on the label. The default is petroleum based. Spectrum is my preferred choice of oil brands. The brands listed in Appendix C (Preferred Brands) use expeller pressed oils and no hydrogenated oils in their products.

Third, *eliminate or minimize the "whites."* The "white" includes white sugar and its aliases (such as brown sugar, cane sugar, corn fructose, corn sweetener, corn syrup, dextrin, dextrose, fructose, fruit fructose, glucose, high fructose corn syrup, invert sugar, lactose, maltose, mannitol, raw sugar, sorbitol, and sucrose). It also includes white flour and its aliases (such as bleached flour, enriched flour, and wheat flour), which work in the body similarly to white sugar. White rice has had its nutrients stripped from it and also works in a similar way in the body to white sugar.

Replace white sugar with more natural sweeteners. Raw, unfiltered honey, pure maple syrup, black strap molasses,

Sucanat (dehydrated cane juice with the minerals), FruitSource (made from rice and grapes), brown rice syrup, and date sugar reflect the many sugar alternatives. *Lifestyle for Health* cookbook tells you how to use each of these and how to troubleshoot using them in your own family favorite recipes.

White flour can be replaced with whole grains. This includes whole wheat, spelt, barley, rice, quinoa, millet, and amaranth. The brands listed in Appendix C utilize these whole grains and produce tasty products.

White rice can be replaced with brown rice. Many people think they do not like brown rice because they have only tasted mushy brown rice or they think it has to take an hour. Lundberg Farms has a great quick brown rice. To cook brown rice to produce a fluffy grain, use the following method:

- Sauté 1 cup brown rice in a small amount of oil (the good kind) until lightly browned. Add 2 cups water and bring to a boil. Cover, lower heat, and simmer, covered for one hour. Remove from heat and let set for about 10 minutes.

Aspartame (NutraSweet) is also not recommended for human consumption. Some scientific research says that there are no "proven" side effects to aspartame. However, every person I have met in the holistic health care arena spurns aspartame even more than white sugar, which is a known health problem.

Fourth, *eliminate or minimize meat, especially those grown with antibiotics, steroids, and hormones*. We do not eat meat in restaurants. The few times we do eat meat we ensure that it comes from a natural source. I recommend Coleman for beef, Shelton's for poultry, and wild meat (such as buffalo, venison, and elk). The taste is far superior without the added chemicals.

Fifth, *eliminate or minimize dairy products*. Dairy is known for its production of mucus in the body. This impacts ear infections, sinus infections, runny noses, and other respiratory problems. Many options exist for this food. Rice, soy, or almond milk work fine in cooking and baking with virtually no noticeable differences. Brands can be found in Appendix C.

Excellent soy and almond cheeses are available that melt well and work fine in casseroles, ethnic dishes, and on pizza. Rella is the brand that I have found melts the best with an excellent flavor.

If you choose to use dairy products, I highly recommend using brands that use organic milk or milk without the bovine growth hormone. Although the effects of this hormone is controversial, we have decided not to give our daughter milk that has growth hormones. Alta Dena, Brown Cow, Cascadian, and Stonyfield Farm are excellent brands for this type of dairy.

Sixth, *minimize the use of canned vegetables and fruits.* Canning removes the most nutrients of any preserving process. The next best step is frozen, then dehydrated. The best choice is fresh. When fresh produce is not available, frozen is preferred over canned.

When purchasing tomato products, I recommend purchasing either those in glasses, boxes, or enamel-lined cans. When tomato products are placed in tin cans, the acid in the tomatoes reacts with the aluminum in the cans. This causes an acidic flavor. It is that flavor that usually requires sugar to be added to recipes. Using a brand such as Muir, which uses enamel-lined cans, eliminates this acidic taste. (Additionally, Muir uses only organic tomatoes.)

STEP 10: LEARN ALTERNATIVES.

The key to getting healthier is not deprivation leading to a bleak future. Rather, the key is knowing the various alternatives for our favorite standbys. In Chapter 11 (20 Common Foods and Their Healthier Alternatives), you will learn of your options for your child's favorite foods. Knowing satisfying options to replace unhealthy foods will encourage your children that you are not trying to deprive them. A feeling of deprivation leads to rebellion and great frustration for you as the parent.

A project as all-encompassing as changing your family's health is made up of many components. Knowing how to divide that large task into smaller units and conquering it one step at a time makes it a doable job. The easiest step to implement is knowing alternatives for the least healthy foods in your kitchen. Parts 3 and 4 are designed to teach you those alternatives. Changing one unhealthy food at a time is an example of effectively "dividing and conquering" the adventure of getting healthy.

STEP 11: HAVE INCENTIVES.

As with any goal, incentives make the journey more fun. Instead of using food as your reward system, develop family interests to use as incentives. Many adult food problems are rooted in childhood food rewards. Avoid creating those problems by not using food as a reward.

Peter Daniels, well-known Australian entrepreneur, says, "It is an absolute fact that without incentives we soon tire and energy is dissipated." Our incentives can be either tangible or intangible. The key is to associate your incentive with the attainment of a specifically predefined goal.

When you do well for "X" period of time (i.e., a week or a month), take time for an outing. Maybe your child would like to go to the library, have an evening of games, or go on a picnic. Maybe you will decide to go hiking, skiing, or for an afternoon walk. The possibilities are endless. And your child will have had some extra time with his/her favorite person — *you.*

STEP 12: REJOICE!

How exciting! You are on the road to better health for you and your child. You are learning how to pass on an inheritance to help build the destiny of your child. Money alone can never buy what you are learning how to provide. I applaud your commitment and say, "Well done."

Don't stop reading, learning, or implementing what you know. The benefits of a healthy lifestyle continue to get better. This is especially true for the child with 70, 80, or 90 "healthy" years ahead. Rejoice, you helped create that future!

SUMMARY OF WHERE TO START

☆ STEP 1: Make A Decision

☆ STEP 2: Get in Unity

☆ STEP 3: Include Your Children

☆ STEP 4: Examine Your Food Traditions

☆ STEP 5: Identify the Cost of Change

☆ STEP 6: Establish the Price You Are Willing To Pay

☆ STEP 7: Develop an Attitude

☆ STEP 8: Begin to ADD
- ••• Add more fruits and vegetables
- ••• Add more organic
- ••• Add more whole grains, beans, raw nuts, seeds, and sprouts
- ••• Add more pure water
- ••• Add supplementation

☆ STEP 9: Begin to SUBTRACT
- ••• Minimize foods processed with chemicals
- ••• Minimize foods with hydrogenated fat pruducts.
- ••• Minimize the "whites"
- ••• Minimize meats with chemicals
- ••• Minimize dairy products
- ••• Minimize canned foods

☆ STEP 10: Learn Alternatives

☆ STEP 11: Have Incentives

☆ STEP 12: Rejoice

—☆—

CHAPTER FOUR

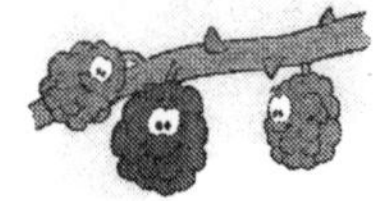

"How can I introduce healthier food to my children without rebellion?" is the question for a smart parent.

Strategies by Age

How can you introduce healthier food without rebellion? That is the question of a smart parent. Health is irrelevant, if in the introduction process, you create rebellion and rigid resistance. At that point you have only added to your problems but not to your solutions.

It is possible to introduce the subject of health and prompt interest, excitement, and momentum. However, those approaches take careful thought, planning, and implementation. In this chapter we will look at strategies that have worked for us and many other families. Our strategies are broken out by age groups. They are in no way meant to be all-inclusive nor are they meant to be prescriptions or replacements for work being done with your health care provider.

PRIOR TO CONCEPTION

An infant's potential for health is predetermined by the collective genetic pool of his/her ancestral family (barring a miracle from God, which is possible).[1] The health of the parent at the time of conception truly impacts the health of the infant and future adult. This health includes physical, mental, emotional, spiritual, and financial.

I was unaware of many of my health conditions prior to the birth of our daughter. So, many of our daughter's health "opportunities" came from my health condition at her conception. So many of those issues could have been avoided, had I taken the time to analyze my state of health and then do something about it.

If you are considering having a child, you are in a marvelous place. You have the opportunity to make an investment in the health of your future children. Do not take this opportunity lightly. It will reap rewards money can never replace or buy.

Prior to conceiving a child, take the time to evaluate your health by asking yourself the pre-conception questions starting on page 78. They are intended to help you explore your philosophy of health and how it impacts an infant prior to the baby's appearance. The questions that leave you stumped give you the opportunity to think. Thinking in advance of a crisis gives you the power of choice. A crisis often leads to rash decisions you later regret. Your answers can help you build a lifetime health strategy that will create a strong child from conception through adulthood.

PREGNANCY

The pregnancy test comes back positive. Now a flood of emotions appear on stage. A baby… your baby. How can you build on your health to create the healthiest baby possible?

---

[1] Mark Percival, *Infant Nutrition,* Health Coach Systems International, Inc. (New Hamburg, Ont., 1991), 1.

During pregnancy, the baby is totally dependent upon the mother's diet and environment. Everything the mother ingests or is even exposed to can effect the baby. Since the baby is so much smaller, these can effect the baby in a much stronger way than it affects the mother.

Because of the hormonal changes in a woman, many dormant health issues may begin to surface during pregnancy. This fact certainly proved true for me. It has taken me nearly ten years to erase the effects of a difficult pregnancy caused by my pre-pregnant state of health.

What can you do to improve your health during pregnancy? The following tips are general. Your particular application of the general tips needs to be customized based on your current status and your goals. Work with a quality health care provider to help you develop a plan that will help produce a healthy birth and child.

Pregnancy Strategies:

1. EXERCISE

From deep breathing to strengthening of the uterus, to stretching, to cardiovascular strengthening, you will benefit from an increase in exercise. Your flexibility, strength, and endurance are greatly needed during the delivery process. A 10 – 15 minute regular exercise routine will help keep you in shape.

Whenever possible, get fresh air, sunshine, and outdoor exercise. The vitamin D from the sun and the oxygen all help add to the strength and health of your body. A daily walk increases flexibility, oxygen, and endurance. Wear flat shoes that provide good support. Check with your health care provider before starting any exercise routine. Anne Charlish and Linda Hughey Holt, MD in Birth Tech (*Tests and Technology in Pregnancy and Birth, Facts on File*, NY, NY, 1991) have many excellent exercise suggestions and cautions.

2. FOOD AND BEVERAGE CHOICES

The food you eat at this time builds the reserves in your child that lays the groundwork for future health. Here are a few general tips for healthier food choices at this time.

- Increase consumption of fruits and vegetables.
- Increase consumption of whole grains, seeds, and sprouts.
- Decrease or eliminate consumption of meat (especially commercial meats with chemicals).
- Eat calcium-rich foods (such as almonds, dark green leafy vegetables, yogurt, asparagus, kale, tofu, brewer's yeast, and sea vegetables).
- Increase iron-rich foods (such as fish, eggs, and leafy green vegetables, such as spinach).
- Drink lots of pure water.
- Decrease refined carbohydrate intake (i.e., desserts, chips, ice cream, refined sugar, etc.).
- Decrease or eliminate caffeine consumption, including cola drinks.
- Eliminate smoking and alcohol consumption.
- To easily add 11.5 mg. of iron and 33.5 mg. of protein to your day, add (for vegetarian diets) 2 Tbl. of brewer's yeast, 1 1/2 cups of soy milk, 1 banana, and 1 oz. of pumpkin seeds.

3. SKIN BRUSHING

Brushing the skin helps stimulate the movement of lymph fluids throughout the body. Lymph is the primary component for all body fluids and hormones. When you stimulate the lymph fluid, you increase nutritional flow in the body.

A natural bristle brush is best for skin brushing. They can be found in health food stores and bath shops. Brushing prior to a shower or bath loosens dead skin. The water from the shower washes this dead skin away. Brush in small, circular motions starting at the body extremities (i.e., feet, hands, and head). Brush toward the heart.

4. MINIMIZE EXPOSURE TO CHEMICALS

Setting up a nursery usually involves painting, new fabrics, and new carpet — all of which contain highly toxic formaldehyde and other "hydes." Our family uses an organic zeolite rock called Natural NonScents to remove those toxins easily and inexpensively. Call our Lifestyle for Health office at 303-771-9357 for more information on where to find this product.

Families have told us of losing or nearly losing their babies due to a "brand new" nursery. The chemical fumes led to many health problems that could have been easily avoided by environmental cleansing prior to moving a new baby home.

X-rays during pregnancy should only occur under exceptional circumstances. This includes dental and medical. When X-rays are necessary, consider wearing a leaded abdominal shield to protect the baby.

Lead pollution, in the form of vehicle pollution, has been linked to low birth weight and impaired development of speech, memory, learning, and intelligence. Try commuting during off-peak hours. Or, consider gentle detox baths by using Epsom salts in a warm bath. Check with your health care provider on this and other cleansing activities during pregnancy.

5. MINIMIZE DRUG USE

Minimize OTC drug use. Be careful with the use of herbs. Each of these forms of medication can impact a baby. Recreational drugs harm an embryo, too. No responsible adult would continue the use of these drugs during pregnancy. Consult your health care practitioner before using any OTC drug or herb.

On the positive side, herbs such as raspberry leaves can strengthen the uterus and be of help during pregnancy. A holistic health care provider can guide you in making helpful herbal choices.

6. MINIMIZE EMOTIONAL STRESS

Obviously emotional and any other form of stress impacts the baby. As much as possible take a mellow attitude to daily stressors. Your getting upset and stressed does not help you or your baby. Get a support team to help build your emotional stamina. Get involved in a local church or women's ministry. Or, include your husband or extended family in deciding how they can specifically support you (and your baby) during this exciting time.

7. MORNING SICKNESS, HEARTBURN AND CONSTIPATION

Some women find milk, yogurt, fruit, or salads to help morning sickness. Herb teas, such as peppermint, linden, and chamomile, can also be very soothing.

Eating smaller meals more frequently may be of help in combatting heartburn. Follow good food combining techniques to help minimize digestive problems. (See my book *Food Smart!* for more information on food combining.) Sprouting legumes and nuts (soaking in water for 24 hours and then draining before using or eating) can make those foods more digestible. Taking digestive enzymes may also help minimize heartburn. Contact the Lifestyle for Health office at 303-771-9357 for information on digestive enzymes.

Constipation can be reduced by increasing water intake, adding high fiber foods (i.e., whole-grain breads, legumes, nuts, fresh produce). Buckwheat is considered a natural remedy for hemorrhoids and also for varicose veins and may also be found to be helpful.

BIRTH THROUGH AGE 1

At this time, a child is highly dependent upon the mother for its nutrition. If the mother chooses to make poor food choices, both the mother and the child will bear the consequences.

Obviously, the best source of nourishment is breast milk (if the mother has a healthy diet). Human milk offers an excellent balance of nutrients and protection. Even the best formula is inferior to breast milk. A powerful antibody (IgA) is found in breast milk, which protects the infant's bowels from bacterial infection. Breast- feeding an infant for a minimum of 6 months greatly reduces incidences of infection and food allergies. There is a consensus that introducing solid foods earlier than 6 months can cause problems.

Introducing solid foods too early bears these potential risks:

- Overfeeding with excessive weight gain and risk of life-long obesity.
- Inadequate neuromuscular maturation, with problems in swallowing, regurgitation, danger of aspiration and choking, difficulty digesting solid foods, along with abdominal pain, diarrhea, gas, and risk of bowel surface damage.
- Risk of inducing allergic responses to food. Absorption of large molecules from the bowel may trigger a variety of delayed allergic responses like eczema, bronchitis, or asthma, and may expose the infant to a high risk of immune-complex disease with serious target organ damage and life-long food allergy.

Food Introduction Strategies

Solid foods should be introduced slowly and pureed. Introduce new foods one at a time over a weekly interval. One new food per week allows the mother to detect any immediate or delayed reactions. Start with one teaspoon in quantity and increase as the infant becomes accustomed to the food. Try one new food for several days before introducing the next food. This will help you determine any allergic reactions more quickly.

The following chart indicates a recommended process for introducing solid foods.

6 MONTHS

Introducing solid foods before 4 to 6 months can negatively impact the immature digestive system, encouraging allergic reactions. The small amount of foods given at this age is basically introducing the baby to the taste and feel of solid foods. Nourishment is still primarily from breast milk (or formula).

Food	**Preparation Method**
Carrots	Scrape, boil until tender. Puree with enough water to make a soft consistency.
Apples	Use sweet apples and no sweetener. Peel, core, slice, and cook in enough water until tender.
Bananas	Use very ripe bananas. Peel and mash, adding water if needed to make a soft consistency.
Avocados	Mash and add water to make a soft consistency.
Zucchini	Cut into small pieces and steam until tender. Puree.
Pears	Same as apples.
Pumpkin	Peel, remove seeds, chop and steam until tender. Puree.
Peaches, Apricots, Nectarines,	Use only very ripe fruit. Remove skin, pits and mash thoroughly.

Plums, Mangoes, Papaya, Kiwi, Sweet Cherries	
Broccoli, Cauliflower, Cabbage	Steam until tender. Puree. If gas occurs, add pureed carrot.
Potatoes	Bake or boil. Mash pulp. May be softened with rice or soy milk.
Corn, Peas, Green Beans	Use fresh or frozen, as canned has added salt and sugar. Cook and puree.

Suggested Feeding Pattern for 6 Month Olds

waking	breast milk
breakfast	breast milk
mid-morning	diluted real fruit juice
lunch	1/2 to 2 tsp. fruit or vegetable puree breast milk
mid-afternoon	diluted fruit juice (unless given in the morning)
dinner	breast milk
bedtime	breast milk

6 TO 8 MONTHS

As solid food intake increases, the baby will demand less breast milk. Your milk supply will follow this decreased demand. There may be a lag time of a couple of months, but it is only temporary. Vegetarian protein additions can now be added to the fruit and vegetable purees.

Food	Preparation Method
Lentils	Make into a thick soup. Can add a vegetable puree.
Beans	Use homecooked, mashed beans. Thoroughly mash and puree. Do not add canned beans until after 8 months.
Nuts, Seeds	Finely mill into a powder consistency with a food processor or thoroughly cleaned seed or coffee grinder. Use a variety of nuts and stir into purees, starting with 1/2 teaspoon.
Wheat Germ	Sprinkle over vegetable purees.
Yogurt	Choose an active plain yogurt with no preservatives or honey. Add to fruit purees, mashed bananas, and powdered nuts.
Eggs	Start with the yolk. When added to hot vegetable puree, the heat will cook the beaten yolk. Later try scrambled eggs. Do not introduce eggs before 18 to 24 months if there is any history of allergies, eczema, or asthma in the family.
Amazake	This is a rice milk made from the whole grain. It can be diluted half and half with pure water or added to baby rice cereals.

Suggested Feeding Pattern for 6 to 8 Month Olds

waking	breast milk
breakfast	baby rice cereal, amazake, or fruit puree breast milk
mid-morning	diluted real fruit juice
lunch	1 to 2 tablespoons of fruit puree, vegetable, lentil, or bean puree breast milk

mid-afternoon	diluted real fruit juice (unless given in the morning)
dinner	same as breakfast breast milk
bedtime	breast milk

8 TO 12 MONTHS

At this age, children will begin to want to eat what the family is eating (is the rest of the family eating healthy?). Be sure the child's portions are not highly seasoned or salted. Many times the family's food can be placed into a blender with a little water and blended for a quick, nutritious meal. Extras can be frozen in ice cube trays for quick "instant" meals.

Suggested Feeding Pattern for 8 to 12 Month Olds

waking	water or diluted real fruit juice
breakfast	oatmeal, baby rice cereal, whole grain bread
mid-morning	diluted real fruit juice
lunch	mashed legumes with vegetables, fruit puree with yogurt, or a vegetable puree water, rice, or soy milk
mid-afternoon	diluted real fruit juice. finger foods of fruits, vegetables, or whole grain crackers.
Dinner	whole grain bread with nut butter or lentil spread, scrambled egg, soups, etc.
Bedtime	breast milk

☆ A blender is an excellent tool to convert steamed vegetables and fruits into pureed soups or sauces (with a little added water). Freshly prepared juices are more tolerable than their commercial counterparts.

☆ Organic baby foods (i.e., Earth's Best) are far superior to many commercially available baby foods. Homemade baby food is cheaper and quite simple with the use of a blender. Blend any food prepared for the family (minus the salt and seasonings). Freeze extra in ice cube trays. Remove the solid cubes, label, and use later for "instant" baby food.

☆ By 9 months, food mixtures can contain some lumps to encourage chewing. By 12 months, food can be well cooked, or raw, and cut into small manageable pieces. One-year-olds are capable of feeding themselves and will have food preferences. It is critical for the parent to develop the "vegetable habit" at this age.

☆ Often infants will reject a new food due to smell or taste. Try mixing a small quantity of this new food with a favorite food. Slowly increase the amount of the new food until the child is eating the new food acceptably. If a child still rejects the new food, there could be an adverse reaction and the new food should be eliminated for the next several weeks. The child is not remembering this food. His brain is reacting to the taste or smell of the food. This is not a conscious decision or "attention getter" at this age. It is a physical reaction to the food.

☆ During this first year, avoid salt and salty foods, such as chips, soy sauce (tamari), and stocks. These foods, along with spices, can add strain to the liver and kidneys. Refined white flour products often contain additives and chemicals. One hundred percent whole grain products may be too high in fiber content for children under 12 months of age. Refined sugar products (i.e., jam, syrups, sweetened juices, etc.) contain only calories with proportionately few, if any, nutrients. The refined sugar is too quickly taken into the blood stream, causing the body to produce large amounts of insulin. Over an extended period of time, this can lead to pancreas dysfunction and diabetes. In addition, honey is not recommended as a safe alternative before 12 months of age.

☆ Processed, canned, and packaged foods with additives, colorings, chemicals, and preservatives are not recommended for children (big or little!). Additives have been linked to hyperactivity and other behavioral and health problems. Whole nuts should not be given to children under age five. They can stick in a child's throat and cause choking. Chocolate, tea and other caffeine products are stimulants and should be avoided. Deep fried foods are hard to digest and undesirable in a baby's diet.

☆ Avoid cow's milk. Cow's milk is in the top two or three common food allergies, for children and adults. It is the major contributor to infant middle ear infections. Milk allergies can cause gastroenteritis, which affects 5–10% of children under 2. Gastroenteritis is an inflammation and irritation of the digestive system, which can result in anemia. Milk allergies can manifest in asthma, eczema, headaches, arthritis, chronic upper respiratory infections, congestion, bronchitis, pneumonia, bed-wetting, so-called growing pains, fatigue, hyperactivity, and even epilepsy in children who have allergy-related migraines.

AGE 1 TO 3 (TODDLERS)

As children move from the first year of life, their own unique tastes and preferences strengthen. If a child has never had junk food, keeping on track is a much easier matter. However, for parents who are just now learning the importance of nutritional food, change can require a little more effort. Here are a few strategies that we have found to be helpful. Many of these strategies are foundational for later ages. It is never too early to begin teaching and implementing health in a child's life.

1. Don't *Nag*.

Even toddlers do not want to constantly be told to eat this or that. Make a decision as to how your family will eat. Be firm and stick to the decision. Give your child what you have decided and do not give into tantrums or other emotional-wrought demands. Given time, even the most "independent" toddler will enjoy healthier foods.

2. Be in *Unity*!

It is amazing how even toddlers figure out when parents, and/or other family members are in disagreement on an issue. If a child goes from one parent to another (especially in split custody situations), the child will quickly identify where the parents disagree. If one parent is pursuing health and the other doesn't care, the child will quickly learn how to drive a bigger wedge via the use of food.

The serious impact is on the child's health. Going from healthy food to junk food plays havoc on the child's body and immune system. It is far better for the parents to come into agreement and be consistent than fluctuate back and forth. Take the time, value your child, and come into unity on the issues of health and food. Even if it will take a few months or years to be able to pursue health to the degree that you would like, don't put the child in the middle of your problems. Emotional health from a family in unity is as critical as physical health from proper nutrition. Don't turn meal time into a war zone, which will antagonize everyone's digestion and ultimate health.

3. Set the *Example.*

Toddlers are great mimickers. They copy what they see, hear, and feel. Don't bother to tell your child to eat vegetables and then skip yours. By the time your toddler is 3, he/she will notice the double standard and call you on it.

As a parent you have the responsibility and privilege to set an example of excellence or mediocrity. The standard you set becomes the standard your child will adopt, knowingly or not. We see abused children grow into adults who abuse. It isn't that they want to abuse. It is that until they are exposed to a different model of behavior, abuse is the only behavior they understand. If you set the example of junk food and health problems, your children will live out that model, until they are taught something else.

4. Make Eating *Fun.*

Keeping mealtimes relaxed and fun is crucial for good digestion and assimilation of nutrients. Instead of talking health, make food fun. Talk about the color of food if the child is learning colors. Have a "green" day and let the child pick whatever "green" food she/he wants to eat. Make flash cards of fruits and vegetables and let your child select favorites while learning the names. Set different produce items out on the counter or table while you are cooking. Let the child place the flash cards next to the same fruit (or vegetable). You are teaching recognition concepts as well as nutritional information.

Let your child pick out a new food at the grocery store for a meal. Kids love to be a helper at this age. Let them pick. Build towers out of carrot circles or build a road out of celery sticks. Cut vegetables can present a wealth of building material to an active imagination. What a far better activity than just watching a video or television. Plus cleanup is a snap, when the toddler can devour the "building materials."

When going for walks or playing outside, have a plate of healthy snacks all ready for your return. Use fun plates or bowls, so that as the child eats the food, a favorite character appears. Taking a few minutes to plan ahead can make eating fruits and vegetables a fun process for you and your toddler.

5. Make It *Look Good!*

Just as adults do, toddlers eat with their eyes. If you have always served junk food, the perception of what "looks good," may need to change. If they are accustomed to lots of candy, sugar-based beverages, and other prepared food items, it will take some time for them to prefer natural foods and beverages. This will require that you truly make a family decision and are in complete unity. The toddler will fairly quickly come around to the new way of eating.

Take the time to put food on a plate. Ages 2 and 3 are not too early to teach eating off of a plate. The children I have known who were allowed to eat off a table or high chair without the benefit of a plate invariably became messy eaters throughout their childhood. It takes a little more time (and patience) to teach the child to eat from a plate, but it is possible. The maternal rewards for a child who eats tidily (in less daily cleanup) far outweighs the time spent teaching the child how to accomplish it.

Put lots of color on a child's plate. Have green at each meal. Don't serve an all white meal. How boring! Add some green, some red, some orange, or yellow. Color will make the food so much more inviting, not to say more nutritious (the deeper the color, the more nutrition!).

6. Be *Consistent*!

It is important to determine a standard that can be maintained at home, at grandparents (and other extended family homes), at friends' houses, and even in restaurants. A lack of consistency here will cause confusion for the child. It will also teach a child to use food as a wedge between authority figures and as a demand-based tool.

So often a parent chooses to eat healthy, yet the grandparents want to continue feeding their new grandchild less than healthy foods (although this can also work in reverse). Take the time to work out these differences of opinion. The more consistent the eating patterns of the child in every area of life at this stage, the healthier the child will be.

AGE 4 TO 5 (PRESCHOOL)

As children reache pre-school age, they are often around other children. If your child is home full-time, as in homeschool families, you are in an excellent position. You have the opportunity to more fully control the food in your child's life. Be sure to take advantage of this opportunity by giving healthy food as often as possible.

If you are dealing with a preschool or other outside child care program, you have several things to consider. The following strategies can be of help in these child care situations and for general resistance by the child to healthier food.

1. *Monitor* Child Care Food Choices.

Traditional snacks at child care centers are usually horrible by any definition (or at least by mine!). Take the time to provide your child with the healthiest snacks you can. If the center is serving milk and graham crackers, have an alternative (i.e., rice milk and whole grain crackers, fresh fruit, or vegetables). Lunches are usually no better. Consider sending a homemade, home-packed lunch with your child.

The best solution is to get the center committed to eating healthy as a group. When the center and/or several parents are interested in health, the problems shrink drastically. Have the center contact our Lifestyle for Health office for information on wholesale health food products in their area (303-771-9357).

2. Offer *Variety*.

Keep your pantry and refrigerator stocked with multiple choices of food. Variety allows for food rotation, which is helpful to prevent any future allergies. It also gives the child many choices, which is a teaching tool in and of itself. This includes variety in produce (especially between seasons), nuts, seeds, cereals, pasta, and breads.

3. Offer *Alternatives.*

If a child is around other children at all, he/she will be exposed to junk food in at least one of its many forms. Having an alternative to highly refined sugar snacks is critical. This doesn't mean just celery sticks or a chunk of tofu! If your child is eating healthy at meals and not eating chips, candy, and soda throughout the day, then a healthier alternative helps the process stick at this age.

For example, instead of sugar-based candy, try sweets made from whole sweeteners without food dyes, additives, and other chemicals (see Preferred Brands for more detail — examples include Sunspire Drops instead of M&M's, Tropical Source for candy bars). Instead of sodas, mix quality, real fruit juices with a carbonated mineral water or a fruit-based spritzer, such as Knudsen's brand. Try using carob-based products instead of chocolate to minimize the caffeine intake. Dried fruits can be used in place of sweet candies. Instead of high fat chips, try some of the new baked chips (Garden of Eatin' has some that actually taste good), whole grain pretzels, popcorn, or nuts (soaked whole almonds are easier to digest and are quite high in calcium).

4. Do Not Use Food for Rewards.

Many parents will offer food as a reward for behavior at this stage. ("Mommy will give you a cookie if you are good.") Many teen and adult eating disorders stemmed from food being used as a reward system. Let food be used for nourishment. Separate behavior and rewards from food. A reward can be time spent with the parent, but not the food itself.

5. Consider *Supplementation.*

In our toxic world, it is usually helpful to consider some type of supplementation at the advice of your health care provider. Appendix B covers specific supplementation suggestions by age. Be sure to check any supplementation with your health care provider.

6. Get *Exercise*.

Chapter 8 discusses physical fitness by age groups. Although many parents believe their children are active and never sit still, the fact is most children are physically inactive in areas that produce overall physical fitness. Even at this early age, encourage your child to get outside, go to parks, and get planned physical activity. Limit or eliminate television viewing, which minimizes physical activity and introduces children to junk food. Developing a family plan in the area of physical activity and television viewing is critical at this age. Make commitments today that you will keep. It is much harder to break habits in the future than to set and keep commitments today, at early ages.

AGE 6 TO 10 (SCHOOL AGE)

Whether your child is homeschooled, in private school, or public school, this age is beginning to explore and develop their own opinions. This is the best time to teach instead of just telling your child what to do. The following strategies can help make that an easier process for you.

1. Let Them *Help*.

At this age, most kids want to be a helper, especially if there is a good parent-child relationship. Encourage them, let them help make up the grocery list, shop, or even begin to cook. Our daughter began making "fruit salads" at the tender age of 5. Since we are frequently involved in hospitality, she "presented" the salad to our guests on a tray complete with little toothpicks for serving. She was so proud of her creation, she suggested I use it in a newsletter.

Since children at this age want to help, let them. Find cookbooks for children (see Appendix A), cooking classes for children, or create your own. Teach your child how to measure. Setting some flour or vegetables with measuring spoons and cups on a table (covered, of course) can entertain for hours. As they learn to measure, they can take the next step and make simple muffins, pancakes, or other recipes. Giving them healthy ingredients teaches them without them being aware of it.

2. Plan for *Peer Pressure.*

If your child is at school away from home or around other children at all, he//she will be exposed to junk food in many forms. This can range from sugar-laden birthday cakes at parties, sweets at Sunday school, junk food at grandparents, or fast food at friends' homes. Children need to be taught how to handle these situations before they are in them. Just as we teach our children not to enter the car of a stranger, we need to teach them how to handle peer pressure regarding food.

We talk to the parents, teachers, and other adults in our child's life. As much as possible we have prepared them with our family's approach to health. As a result we have limited Anna to many difficult situations. However, the pressure is still there. Where possible, we let her pick her healthier alternatives to take to parties and friends' homes. I always send enough for everybody to try some, so she can be a giver and include the other kids. When possible I accept the responsibility to provide the food in social gathering. Yes, it is more work, but it gives us control of the food that is available.

3. Teach *Choices* and *Consequences.*

As parents, Forest and I have committed to teaching Anna that she has the responsibility to make choices. We help her, but we also have helped her learn how to make choices. We play games of "what if." For example, we discuss what happens to her friends that eat junk food all of the time (they are usually frequently sick). We point out how children smell who come from homes where parents smoke. We discuss children with behavior problems who eat massive amounts of sugar. By the ages of 8 and 9, she was beginning to see the cause and effect of food in other children's lives.

The few times that Anna has chosen to eat junk food and has experienced some type of physical consequence, we talk about it. We don't condemn or judge, we discuss consequences of choices. We ask what would have been a better choice. Together we determine how we could prevent a repeat of the current problem and identify several possible solutions. This is teaching her how to be responsible for her body and its health. As she learns responsibility in the area of food at this age, appeal of the temptation to smoke, do drugs, or have premarital sex is greatly diminished during the teen years. Teaching principles and the responsibility of choice at this age pays great rewards as the child gets older. This lays a strong foundation for adult responsibility.

4. Make *Tasty* Food.

Nothing is worse than "blah" health food. One of the reasons I have included recipes in this book is to help you introduce *tasty* healthy food to your family. I have several other healthy cookbooks available. I began writing cookbooks when I observed how dull, tasteless, and ugly many health food recipes were. I am a firm believer that health food should look better and taste better than any other type of food. If the food doesn't taste good, it doesn't matter how healthy it is, nobody, especially a child at this age, will eat it. Learn how to make your health food choices taste good. Learn which brands provide tasty alternatives (see Appendix C).

5. Be *Prepared.*
We never leave home without a healthy snack and pure water. So many times, our "quick" trip turned into a several-hour activity. Children at this age are frequently hungry. Having a health snack available can avoid many temptations to drop by for fast food. Having children take their own bottles of pure water gives them a healthier option to soda machines that are so readily available.

AGE 10 TO 18 (PRETEEN AND TEENS)

This age is typically the most challenging, especially if they have not eaten healthy prior to this. Trying to get a teen to change eating habits offers a whole set of "opportunities." However, it is possible and we have heard several success stories to confirm this.

The closer they are to the teen years, the more they want to exercise control to make their own choices. Consequently, in most situations, I have not found it successful to tell teenagers that they can no longer eat foods they have eaten for years. They may obey at home, but the likelihood of rebellion outside of the home is great.

Teens are rarely concerned that they might die of cancer at a later age because most teens are too "now" oriented. Warnings often fall on deaf ears. How can you help motivate teens to make changes in their daily routine to produce health?

1. Don't Make a *Declaration.*
The worst thing you can do is to announce to your family, "We are all going to eat healthy from here on out." Even though you may be excited about your new-found knowledge, your teen will probably look at you with amazement-turning-into-resistance-followed-by-outright rebellion. Consider such ultimatums as a sure-fire way to bring dissension into the home. Don't bother to do it, it won't work.

2. *Communicate.*
If you have chosen to eat healthy for your own reasons, communicate these "I" messages to your teen. If you have experienced health problems and are changing to address these issues, tell your teen. Many teens are quite compassionate and want to understand their parents. If you ask them to help you make these changes, they will often participate as a guise of helping you. They may not be as strict in their implementation as you, but any improvement is an improvement.

3. Make Health *Personal.*
Most teens don't care about cancer from food, smoking, or other sources. So don't bother to try and motivate them with these arguments. Most of all, don't argue. Look for information that is related to areas of interest to your teen. For example, if your teen competes in sports, look for information on physical endurance and performance caused by food. Talk to your daughter about health and skin or PMS. Giving information in an honest, uncritical manner on subjects of interest to them can open many doors that arguing only slams shut.

4. They Learned From *You.*
Remember, your child is a the product (fruit) of what you have already taught him/her. If your teen is not the person you would like, instead of criticizing your son or daughter take a look at your life yesterday. It may be time for you to repent of past parental negligence in the area of food/health. You fed them and taught them to be who they are today. Sincere repentance can also open many doors of communication that have been tightly shut for years.

5. It's Their *Choice.*
You may need to realize that the information you are giving them now may not go into effect for a few years. By the teen

years, they will choose what goes into their mouths and how they will treat their bodies. Be willing to let them also reap the consequences. If the rest of the family has chosen to embrace health food, then, without revenge or other poor attitudes, give them the freedom to join the family or cook their own food. If they cook their own food, they may need to buy it. Develop a plan that doesn't compromise you, yet lets your teens live with the consequences of their choices.

The more you *push* good nutrition, the more your teen will probably rebel. They have no desire to do something that will make them different from their peers, unless they personally have a sense of destiny and direction. If you believe in the power of prayer and personal God, this is a good time to ask for specific wisdom and revelation. Contact our Lifestyle for Health office (at P.O. Box 3871, Littleton, CO 80161). We spend time each Monday praying over written prayer requests.

The following questions are designed to help you work through possible problems at different age levels. Use them as a way to analyze and understand why you are where you are. Once you understand that, the solution often becomes readily apparent. May God bless you with wisdom as you impart health to your children at each stage of their lives!

Pre-conception Questions

1. How did I score on the self-test in Chapter 2? What steps could I take to improve my health in the short term and the long term? Am I willing to do that? Have I (or my spouse) taken birth control pills? Do I know the impact of the pill to my health?

2. What health beliefs am I willing to pass on to my child? Am I willing to nurse? Do I want to vaccinate my child? Will I feed my child formula? Will I feed my child commercial baby food? Will I work with a pediatrician or a pediatric nutritionist? Will I

use chiropractic care with my child? Will I use antibiotics or natural approaches for my child? Ask why or why not with each question.

3. Am I willing to emotionally nourish my child by giving of my personal time? Am I willing to learn who my child is and what gifts God has given this child? Am I willing to help build a family to emotionally nurture my child? What emotional strengths do I have as a future parent? Am I willing to grow emotionally? Ask why or why not with each question.

4. What spiritual beliefs do I have? Do I want my child to have my beliefs? Will my beliefs build a stronger child? How will I teach those beliefs? Why should my child adopt my beliefs? Do I pick the timing of the conception and birth of my child or does God? Ask why or why not with each question.

5. Am I financially responsible? How will I handle the issue of health insurance? Hospital stays? Do I want my child in a hospital? Will I work with a doctor or midwife? Ask why or why not with each question.

Pregnancy Questions

Take at look at your expectations and some of the tough questions that need to be examined.

1. When I think about being pregnant, I feel:

2. I want my child to be:
(i.e., boy vs. girl, smart, tall, attractive, etc.)
Why?

3. I am afraid my child will be:
(i.e., sick, deformed, an intrusion in my life)
Why?

4. My best attributes for being a parent are:
Why?

5. The best possible pregnancy would be:

6. The worst thing that could happen during my pregnancy would be:
What can I do to prevent that?

7. During my pregnancy, I want my husband and family members to help:

8. I expect delivery to be:

9. I expect the first week of my baby's life to look like:
I will need help with:

10. How much time do I or my spouse need to take off during the baby's birth?
Why?

11. Will I have outside child care for my baby?
The qualifications for such help are:

Infant Questions

1. I'm tired, so am I shortchanging my baby of healthy nourishment? What can I do about it?

2. Are my baby's grandparents committed to our family health plan? How will I handle any conflict?

3. How do I presently handle any signs of sickness in my baby? Do I have any other options? What are they? Am I willing to pursue them?
Why or why not?

4. How healthy is my baby?
What do I base that opinion on?

Toddler Questions

1. How often does my child snack? Are his/her snacks supplementing or negatively impacting mealtime?

2. What is it that toddlers like and how can I work with those preferences? Do I have healthy alternatives in my pantry?
Why or why not?

3. What does my child care center believe about health and nutrition? How does that affect me and my child? What can I do about it? Am I willing to make changes?

4. How much regular exercise does my toddler get? Am I part of that exercise plan?

Pre-School Questions

1. Am I connecting food rewards with behavior?

2. How many sweets and refined snacks is my child getting? What are my options?

3. What are my plans to improve the quality of my child's birthday party and holiday food choices?

4. How do I handle resistance by my pre-schooler to health food choices? Are there other options?

School Age Questions

1. Has my child changed eating patterns? Are there signs of eating disorders? Are he/she overly weight conscious?

2. How do the families of my child's friends eat? Have I talked to them about eating healthier?

3. How often do my children participate in preparing meals? How could I include them more? Are they using what I have taught them in making restaurant food choices? Is that good?

4. When was my last discussion of food with my child? Was it positive? Why or why not?

Teen Questions

1. What motivates my teen? How is health tied to that motivation?

2. Do I have open lines of communication with my teen? Why or why not?
Do he/she know why health is important to me at a heart level?

3. What is the real source of conflict between my teen and I? What is the real source of harmony with my teen and I? What do those two answers reveal to me about my role as a parent?
4. What is the most important gift I want to give my teen? Why?
Is a lifetime of health important with that gift?

CHAPTER FIVE

The more you minimize your child's exposure to toxins, the more reserves you are providing for your child.

Extra Lifesavers

In this chapter, we will look at the affects of additives, pesticides, household toxins, and the microwave on the health of your child. Our look will be brief and in summary form. Options will be given and resources for many of these options can be found in the appendices of this book.

The primary damage done by these different entities is in the negative impact to our immune system. As more and more toxins, as well as pollution and poor food choices, become a regular part of children's lives, they will have significant damage done to their immune systems. The consequence is that they will be vulnerable to sickness and disease as a lifestyle. The more you minimize your child's exposure to toxins, the more reserves you are providing your child.

ADDITIVES

Food additives are chemicals added to food to "improve" taste, texture, color, and shelf life. Additives came from the use of salt, smoke, spices, and sugars to preserve foods. Commercial food additives are regulated by governmental agencies. We will quickly look at sulfites, nitrites, salicylates, dyes, and MSG.

Sulfites:
Sulfites are used to bleach and preserve food. They are often diagnosed as allergenic. Symptoms of sulfite allergies include flushing, dizziness, wheezing, or shortness of breath. Sulfite sprays are used on produce and on salad bars. They are often found in wines, beers, and even in drugs. Sulfites are also used to keep the color of dried fruits. Recent governmental regulation has begun to limit their use. Purchasing fresh and dried fruits in health food stores can help limit the intake of sulfites.

Nitrites:
Nitrites, usually sodium salts, are frequently used in bacon and other processed meat (lunch meat, bologna). When they combine with some amino acids in the bowel, they can become carcinogenic. Vitamin C helps to inhibit this reaction. If you choose to eat foods with nitrites, be sure to take extra vitamin C supplementation.

Salicylates:
The grandfather of salicylates is aspirin. Salicylates can also be found in foods and can trigger asthma and has been implicated in deaths due to respiratory failure. Dr. Feingold has done extensive research in the areas of salicylates, allergies, and children's behavioral problems. You can contact the Feingold Organization at 703-768-3287 for more information on salicylates and children.

Food Dyes:
Dyes have often been associated with allergic reactions and behavioral problems in children. Food dyes are used in many

commercial food products. Any item with a number (i.e., #5) in an ingredient list is an example of a food dye. Food coloring used at home is another example. Yellow food coloring has been associated with hives. It is often found in commercial pasta and cookies. Symptoms occurring within 90 minutes of ingesting can include asthma, hives, swelling, headaches, and behavior changes. Safe alternatives are plant-based colors, such as beet juice.

Monosodium Glutamate (MSG):
MSG continues to be a controversial additive. MSG is contained in the food enhancer "Accent." I have found MSG to cause headaches, bloating, and other side effects. With the current labeling regulations, labels must show all ingredients, which would include MSG. Severe sensitivities to MSG can cause shock. MSG sensitivity may indicate a need for B6.

PESTICIDES

The following information will give you a quick overview of the negative impact of pesticides in the life of your child. Alternatives to pesticides follow. According to the Code of Federal Regulations 162.10, it is illegal to claim that a pesticide is safe, even if the label contains a qualifying phrase such as "when used as directed." Children who live in homes in which household and garden pesticides are used have a seven times greater chance of developing childhood leukemia. In a 1983 San Francisco survey, DDT was found to be the most common pesticide residue found on fresh produce. (Although DDT has been banned since 1972, it can still be found on food crops.)

Presumably farmers have added pesticides to reduce insect damage and increase crop production. Yet, interestingly enough, since the use of agricultural pesticides have increased tenfold in the last thirty years, crop losses due to insects have doubled. It is also interesting to note that a pesticide that has been previously banned for use in this country can still be used if the EPA grants an emergency waiver.

Pesticides can remain active for days, weeks, and even years. A common misconception about pesticide applications is that the pesticide is no longer harmful after it has "dried." The fact is that some pesticides have a half life of 50 to 75 years (DDT, for example). Of the 35,000 pesticides used in the U.S., only 10% have been tested. When U.S.-outlawed pesticides are exported, they are used on the foods we import. Typically, imported foods tend to have more pesticides. Most commonly used pesticides in Third World countries are unregistered, banned, or severely restricted in the U.S.

When you simply wash produce (grown with pesticides), nothing happens. Most pesticides are formulated to be water-resistant. Washing all produce in Shaklee Basic H or other commercial produce washers can help pull off some of the oil-based pesticides.

Spraying lawns and for bugs can cause tremendous side effects to children. Not only do the air-borne pollutants pose damage, but so does the leakage into underground water supplies. Since pesticides are designed to impact the "pest's" nervous system, the pesticide will also affect a child's (and adult's) nervous system. Direct contact with these sprayed lawns, through play, can also impact a child.

Pesticide Solutions:

☆ Organic food is grown without the use of chemicals. Technically, the word *organic* is defined in only a few states. In California, *organic* has been defined as food that is "produced, harvested, distributed, stored, processed, and packaged without the application of synthetically compounded fertilizers, pesticides, or growth regulators." This is different from "pesticide-free" labels. "Pesticide-free" indicates that a random inspection of the food was done at the docks and no pesticides were detected at that time. However, half of pesticides applied to crops cannot be detected with these routine tests. Organic food is the purest, most delicious, and nutritious food available.

☆ For alternative, nontoxic pest control, see *Poisoning Our Children*, by Nancy Sokol Green. Another excellent resource is *Bug Busters — Poison-Free Pest Controls For Your Garden*, by Bernice Lifton.

☆ For simple home remedies to pesticides, try the following:

- ••• Diluted cayenne pepper, chili pepper, paprika, or dried peppermint can be used to repel most insects.
- ••• Use mint or lavender to repel ants.
- ••• Spray ants with clove oil diluted in warm soapy water.
- ••• Use garlic and bay leaves to help keep roaches away.
- ••• Make natural flypaper by spreading honey or molasses (thin layer) onto yellow paper.

HOUSEHOLD TOXINS

Household toxins have become so common we often overlook the negative impact on the lives of our children, whose immune systems are quite vulnerable. The number of household toxins continue to increase. I have found that the added load of toxins when traveling (similar to the average home) is as critical as poor food choices in my health. I strongly recommend minimizing as many household toxins in your home as possible. As you eliminate toxins, you will be amazed at how sensitive and aware you will be the toxins in other homes, malls, restaurants, and hotels.

Toxic vapors, such as formaldehyde, can be found in new building and furnishing materials (i.e., particle board and chip board, plywood, carpets, pads, paints, furniture, upholstery foam, plaster, and fabrics). These vapors can take as long as eight to ten years to gas out. In the meantime you suffer from the negative impacts to your immune system in the form of flu-like symptoms, skin lesions, and respiratory problems.

A gas oven cooking at 350 degrees with poor ventilation produces as much carbon monoxide and nitrogen dioxide gas as is in the smoggy skies of Los Angeles (Carikyn Ruben, "Warning: Your Home May be Hazardous to Your Health," *East West Magazine* 10, no. 7 July 1989). If you choose to have a gas oven, be sure it is well ventilated and have it frequently checked for leaks. The same is true for gas fireplaces.

I often thought the reason I was so tired after a day of housecleaning was because I hated to clean. That is true (I do hate to clean), but the bigger contributor was the toxins found in most commercial household cleaners. I have since switched to biodegradable, natural cleaners (I use Shaklee) and have found immeasurable relief. Household cleaning products are among the most toxic substances. Cleaning products are not legally required to disclose everything used in the products. Cleaning products are not regulated by any government agency before coming on the market. Once you omit strong cleaners, even powders such as Comet, from your regular cleaning routine, you will be amazed at how much better your home smells and feels. As you use natural cleaners (including bath soaps, dishwashing liquids, etc.), you will find that you need a less strong cleaner to get the job done. Natural soaps, for example, have minimal, if any, soap buildup.

Sick-building syndrome is not limited to high rise office buildings. It can and does include schools. New, windowless, portable classrooms can easily contain hazardous materials and have little ventilation — two key factors that lead to indoor air contamination. Symptoms from sick-building syndrome can include chronic fatigue, respiratory problems, skin problems, and flu-like symptoms. If your child is in an airtight or new school building, I strongly encourage you to take a look at the following alternatives.

☆ "Gas outs" is when a building/home is completely closed up and the heat is turned up as high as possible. Leave as long as possible, up to a weekend. This intense heat increases outgassing by up to 400% and can reduce overall chemical levels by up to 25%. Thoroughly air the building/home before returning.

☆ Use the product Natural NonScents. Call Nancy Rice at 303-232-2459 for more information. This organic rock (a zeolite) has the ability to adsorb chemicals, odors, and stain. It comes in a rock, powder, or liquid form to be used to remove chemicals with absolutely no odor or perfumes. I have used it in our new home, when I travel, in fruit bowls (slows down fruit ripening), in bathrooms, and in many other ways.

☆ If you are adding new furniture or doing any remodeling in your home or your child's room, seal off as much of the vapors as you can. Apply a nontoxic sealant to the surface of any particle board (i.e., cabinets). Install vapor barriers to keep vehicle fumes from entering a home. Attach vapor barriers to each wall and ceiling leading from the garage to another room on the home. Use as many naturally-occurring elements when building or remodeling a home. Use hardwood floors, tiles, and linoleum where possible. Keep a child's bedroom and play area as toxic-free as possible.

☆ Open windows as much as possible to allow for natural ventilation. However, if pesticides are sprayed anywhere near your home, consider closing windows for a period of time to limit your exposure (realizing that pesticides are still operating even when you can't smell them).

☆ Use natural fiber clothing as much as possible (i.e., cotton, wool, and silk), instead of synthetics. Consider cloth diapers over disposable. The number of chemicals, perfumes, and other toxins in disposable diapers and synthetic fibers is significant. Many diaper covers (i.e., Nikky or Bumpkin) are available. They make changing cloth diapers as easy as disposable. Check the alternative product list found in Appendix C. If you do choose to use disposable diapers, find the ones with the least amount of chemicals.

☆ When purchasing toys, seek those made from natural materials, such as wood and cotton. These toys may cost more to purchase, but they will undoubtedly last longer than their cheaper counterparts. If you choose to get plastic toys (i.e., "Barbie"), let the toy sleep outside to outgas. Store these toys in rooms other than your child's bedroom.

☆ Decorate a nursery as far in advance as possible. Many infant deaths and health crises can be linked to a toxic nursery. Minimize toxic exposure to your newborn, toddler, and child by carefully monitoring all that you let into your home.

MICROWAVES

Microwaves are considered "essential" to the average family. Although most people consider them safe, let me share a few insights. Inside microwaves are "susceptors," which are discs or strips that heat up and brown food. These susceptors contain hazardous chemicals and materials around them that break down in the intense heating process of using the microwave. This creates even more toxins.

The packaging used in microwavable food (i.e., plastics, etc.) can leach dangerous elements into the food. Specially designed plastic wrap has hazardous additives, such as diadipate (2-ethylhexyl or DEHA), which can leach into fatty foods.

Many researchers believe that bacteria such as salmonella and listeria survive the microwaving process. This is especially true if the food has been salted prior to cooking. The more salt the food contains, the more likely the microwaves will not be able to penetrate the center of the food. This creates "cold" spots that do not cook and are susceptible to bacteria growth. The variance caused by these "cold" spots can be as much 60 to 70 degrees.

To avoid these harmful aspects of a microwave, consider not using one (we have found we can live without a microwave). If that is too drastic, consider only using a microwave to reheat food instead of actually cooking. At the very least, do not cook meat, especially poultry, in the microwave. Cooking small, uniform pieces of food, while rotating, will also help minimize the possibility of bacteria growth.

Resource information from:

Nancy Sokol Green, *Poisoning Our Children* (Chicago: Noble Press Inc., 1991).

Part Two:

A Word About Total Health

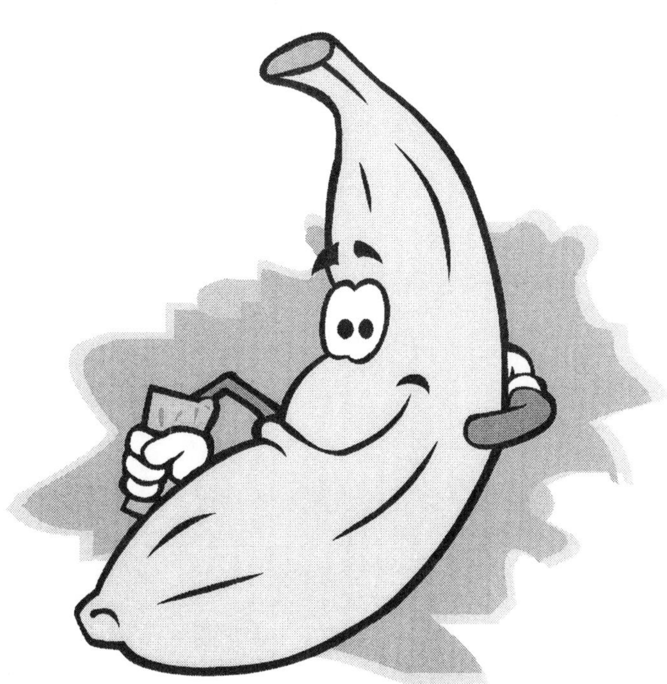

CHAPTER SIX

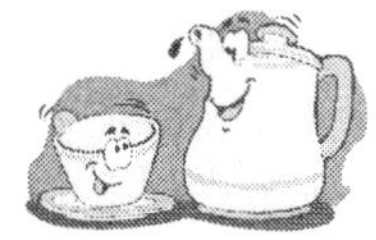

Dispel the myth that nutrition is overwhelming — set nutrition in its proper place — one step at a time.

Let's Explain Nutrition

Many people are overwhelmed at the thought of eating healthier. Somehow our media and conflicting information has caused nutrition to seem mysterious and unobtainable. Let's dispel these intimidating myths and set nutrition in its proper place. Nutritional principles are simple, easy to understand, and can be implemented at many levels.

The real key is effecting nutritional changes one step at a time. If you try and do too much at one time, you can become overwhelmed to the point of paralysis. That is thoroughly ineffective. Take the time to do it one step at a time. Remember, health is a process. Bringing health to your family or your child is a process just as your pregnancy was a process and certainly not instantaneous.

The following principles give you the basics of nutrition. For more information on specific nutrients and their food, see my book *Food Smart!*

NUTRITIONAL PRINCIPLES

1. Get *Educated.*

The most important step in getting you and/or your child healthy is to get educated. So many of my health problems and, consequently, our daughter's came from incorrect information I believed regarding health.

Nourishment is more than poking food into your child's mouth. It means providing nutritious food without chemical or allergenic foods. It includes having variety and proper food preparation. This book will give you many of the basics of good nutrition for your child.

2. *Variety* is the Spice of Life.

One of the easiest ways to avoid allergies is to rotate your foods and provide as much variety as possible. So many Americans tend to eat the same foods day after day. Frequently these foods are craved. This is another indicator of a food allergy (we tend to crave allergenic foods).

Keeping a simple food diary of what you serve your child can help you become aware of the variety, or lack thereof, that you are providing for your child. This diary can also note any reactions he/she might experience. Reactions can indicate allergies or food sensitivities.

It is easy to vary foods throughout the year. Each season offers us different fruits and vegetables naturally. Learn to serve more than corn, peas, and potatoes. Try different greens, different kinds of potatoes, and even new kinds of fruits. The options are almost endless. If you or your child do not like a certain food the first time, don't hesitate to try it once again at a later date. As your body gets healthier, your taste buds will change, too.

3. Eat a *Balance* of Nutrients.

We all know that protein is important. However, too much can actually cause a loss in calcium and other problems. It is possible for children to get enough protein for their growing bones and teeth without ever eating meat. You may not choose to go totally vegetarian (although much research correctly promotes this direction), but you can definitely cut back on commercial meat consumption. Later in this chapter we will look at the content of commercial meats.

Excess protein, found in most American diets, is converted to fat and stored. Red meat and dairy products are not necessary for adequate protein. Beans, peas, vegetables, potatoes, and whole grains provide ample sources of protein. Yogurt, if dairy is tolerated, can also provide protein.

Although research indicates the bulk of our diet should be carbohydrates, carbohydrate consumption has actually decreased by one third over the past fifty years.[1] Not only has our consumption decreased, those carbs that we do eat are usually refined in the form of sugar, candy, white flour, and white rice. The best sources of complex carbohydrates are fresh fruits, fresh vegetables, and whole grains.

Most Americans, especially children, eat nearly twice as much fat as recommended (40% vs. 20%). Most of this fat is the wrong kind, too. Saturated fats are found in meat or animal-based products and need to be minimized or eliminated. Hydrogenated, or partially hydrogenated, fats are also a problem. These include margarines, shortenings, and products using these ingredients. They are virtually indigestible by the body and should be avoided.

---

[1] Jim Braly, *Dr. Braly's Food Allergy and Nutrition Revolution* (New Canaan, CT: Keats Publishing, Inc., 1992), 236.

Children and adults do need essential fatty acids (EFAs) instead of saturated fats and hydrogenated fats. EFAs provide energy. They are also a key component in body tissues and membranes. This impacts the skin, mucous membranes, digestion, and a host of other functions. This means that EFAs help protect the body from anything harmful trying to access it. EFAs also help with numerous metabolic activities including blood pressure, chemical balances, steroid production, appetite and hunger control, and balance of the blood sugar, among others.

Quality sources of EFAs include nuts, seeds, raw vegetables, cold-water fish, and flaxseed oil. We add flax oil to our morning fruit drink for our daily dose of EFAs. We have noticed immediate improvements, especially with our daughter and her health.

4. Know *When* and *How* to Eat.

Feeding children the bulk of their food early in the day can help prevent unnecessary weight gain (this is true for adults, too). Food eaten at night is stored as fat, whereas food consumed throughout the day is used for energy.

The body operates on a schedule, whether we are aware of it or not. That clock leads the body into performing certain activities. That body cycle is shown below.

••• 4:00 a.m. to 12:00 p.m. (noon) Elimination Time

During this time body waste and food debris are eliminated. It is best to eat only fruits or fruit-based drinks during this time. Fruits quickly digest and therefore minimally affect the elimination process.

••• Noon to 8:00 p.m. Appropriation Time

Eating and digestion occur during this time. Fruits, veggies, proteins, and carbohydrates should be eaten during this time.

••• 8:00 p.m. to 4:00 a.m. Assimilation Time

Food is absorbed and used during this part of the cycle. Food should not be eaten at this point.

Encourage your child to eat slowly and to thoroughly chew food. The mouth is the first phase of digestion. Chewing well allows food to become partially digested thereby saving the rest of the digestive system (i.e., the stomach) from excess work. It also helps eliminate indigestion in the form of belching, gas, and bloating.

Take any supplements with meals. Having your child take a supplement on an empty stomach can cause nausea. This can discourage your child from wanting to take supplements.

Do not force your child to clean his or her plate. If they are not snacking unnecessarily and are being fed tasty, healthy food, children are the best indicator of when they are full. Growth spurts cause an increase in hunger and dormant times can cause a decrease in hunger. Do not expect the same hunger level day in and day out.

5. Eat *Raw* Foods When Possible.

It is a startling fact to know that 1 in 4 of our children eat *no* servings of fruits and vegetables a day. Fruits and vegetables are a key source of vitamins and minerals. In their raw form, they are the primary source of enzymes. Enzymes are critical for digestion and unlocking the nutritional value in vitamins and mineral. They play a role in the body similar to spark plugs in a car. Without enzymes, your child won't be going very far!

"Enriched" foods have been so degraded that they have minimal nutritional value to the body. Getting maximum nutrition requires getting some raw foods (i.e., fruits, vegetables, nuts, or seeds) in your child's diet on a daily basis.

Next to raw, it is best if foods are minimally cooked and processed. Excess cooking, refining, and processing strips the food of its nutrients and fiber. Much of the diarrhea and constipation problems of children can be traced back to the intake of primarily processed foods. Fiber is found in whole grain foods, fruits, and vegetables, *if* they are not processed or cooked too much.

6. Avoid *Sugar*.

Over the last 150 years, we have increased our consumption of sugar by more than 100 pounds per year per person. Sugar is a potential allergenic food, highly addictive, and can impact hyperactivity, mood swings, depression, elevated cholesterol, mental and nervous disorders, and diabetes. Your child needs none of these problems.

Refined sugars should be avoided in your child's diet at all times. Check labels as refined sugar can show as sucrose (any "-ose" is questionable), brown sugar, fructose, dextrose, corn syrup, sorbitol, mannitol, and xylitol. You must read labels to know if the food you are buying contains refined sugar. With the introduction of "low fat" and "fat free" products, refined sugar content has soared even higher. The new labels do require the exposure of total carbohydrate dietary fiber coming from sugar.

Since sugar is addictive, you and/or your child will probably notice some withdrawal symptoms when you begin to eliminate sugar from your diet. Withdrawal symptoms might include headaches, irritability, joint aches, digestive upset and cravings. Given a few days those symptoms will disappear. Extra doses of Vitamin C can be helpful in dealing with these symptoms.

The products listed in Appendix C use natural sweeteners. Our *Lifestyle for Health* cookbook has a complete section on refined sugar alternatives and how to use them for food that tastes good.

7. Watch the *Salt*.

Teaching your child to need salt on every dish is unnecessary and potentially harmful. Processed foods often have excess salt or sodium. Our family has found that sea salt (available in health food stores) and Celtic salt are more flavorful and less harmful (for more information, contact the Grain & Salt Society, P.O. Box DD, Magalia, CA 95954, 917-872-5800). Another excellent product is Real Salt or Orsa Salt, which is mined in Utah.

Most people, including children, consume 10 to 50 times more salt than they need. Avoid high-sodium (salt) foods such as processed meats, chips, pretzels — even sweet foods such as soft drinks and sugar-laden jellies. Be especially careful of cheap soy sauces (tamari is much better, free of wheat, and more flavorful), which will cause added thirst due to the high sodium content. San-J is the brand of tamari we prefer. They have an excellent reduced-sodium tamari.

8. Avoid *Dairy* Products.

Most ear infections and many respiratory problems in children stem from dairy consumption. Dairy products are one of the leading allergenic foods. Dairy products are also high in saturated fats.

Signs of dairy intolerance will show as constipation, bloating, abdominal cramping, excess mucus, and respiratory problems. Many excellent dairy substitutes are available. From almond milk to rice milk to soy milk, these alternatives work superbly for cooking and baking. Recipes are included to make these items (Chapter 12) and brands are available for ready-made options (Appendix C).

Alternative cheeses (Rella is a brand I prefer) are available in almond, rice, and soy bases. The Rella brand melts well and most children won't even miss the dairy version. If they do notice, then mix half and half and slowly move toward the dairy-free version.

9. Drink *Water*.

Pure water is critical for the overall health of your child. To determine the needed amount, calculate the following:

- ••• Divide your child's weight by 2 = # of ounces per day of water intake
- ••• Divide ounces by 8 for number of glasses to consume

Water is necessary for overall hydration of the body. Since the body is at least 70% water, a lack of water effects virtually every part of the body, especially the brain. Tap water has numerous contaminants not helpful to a child. We have found distilled or purified (reverse osmosis) water to be the healthiest. This water can be found at health food stores or some supermarkets. Home water filter systems are also available.

10. Minimize the Use of *Antibiotics*.

So many parents reach for an antibiotic at the first sign of sickness. As a result, most children have weakened immune systems. Many childhood problems can be handled without the use of antibiotics. Examples of alternative treatments for common childhood disorders can be found in Chapter 9.

Excess use of antibiotics leads to a loss of the healthy bacteria in the intestinal tract. This often leads to ear infections, yeast (or thrush) infections, and other problems. If antibiotics are taken, be sure to follow with an intake of acidophilus to help restore the friendly bacteria to the gut.

11. Be *Patient*.

It takes time to convert or learn how to become healthy. Give yourself and your child permission to take time. Do not expect either you or your child to be perfect in this process. After working on our health since 1989, we still have a few setbacks. We also continue to learn more about health. The more we learn, the more we realize we have yet to learn.

The body was created to heal itself, given even half a chance. The real miracle is that our children are even alive given what we have done to their environment, food, and bodies. Keep improving and your child's health can be restored. I bless you with patience, encouragement, and the tools to get the job done!

CHAPTER SEVEN

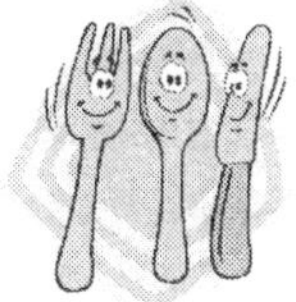

80% of American children are deficient in vitamins and minerals.

Nutritional Requirements by Age

Nutrients are the building blocks of health. As we look at the various vitamins, minerals, and nutrients, we will look at requirements by age, sources, and signs of deficiency. A brief definition will be given in the beginning to give you a working knowledge of the nutrients.

Protein: Protein is the "building block" material for making strong muscles, blood, hormones, hair, fingernails, and immune antibodies. Protein is composed of various amino acids. Amino acids are required by the body and are essential for the healthy growth of a child.

Energy: Your child's body requires "fuel" for energy. Having adequate energy supplies allows the body to concentrate on muscle contraction, nerve impulse conduction, hormone productions, wound repair, cell growth, and a number of other bodily functions. Carbohydrates help utilize energy in the body.

Vitamins: Vitamins serve the function of co-factor for enzymes, which are essential to overall health. Protein production and metabolism are exercised by using these active substances. Enzymes have been called "human spark plugs" and are required for all vitamins to perform their vital chemistry.

Water Soluble Vitamins: These vitamins are not stored in the body and must be consumed every day. This includes vitamins C, B complex, and folic acid.

Fat Soluble Vitamins: These vitamins are stored in the liver and need to be consumed three to five times per week. These include vitamins A, D, E, and K.

Minerals: Earth elements including potassium, sodium, iron, zinc, selenium, calcium, iodine, and chromium are required for electrical and chemical reactions in the body.

Studies indicate that 80% of American children are deficient in vitamins and minerals. Unfortunately, with today's agricultural conditions, it is very difficult for a child to receive the recommended daily allowances without some form of supplementation. See Appendix B for suggested supplementation for various age groups.

SPECIFIC NUTRIENT OVERVIEW

VITAMIN A

Function: A is essential for maintaining membrane tissue and resisting infection in sinuses, lungs, air passages, gastrointestinal tract, vagina, and eyes. It prevents night blindness and oversensitivity to light. Vitamin A also promotes growth, vitality, appetite, and digestion. A helps prevent aging and senility. It helps counteract damaging effect of air pollution.

Sources: dark green leafy vegetables, orange and yellow fruits and vegetables, whole grains, sprouts, seaweed.

Enemies: air pollutants, alcohol, coffee, cortisone, excess iron, mineral oil, lack of sun.

Deficiency Signs: eye, nerve, and lung disorders, sterility, dry-scaly skin, cancer, frequent infections, stunted growth, glandular malfunction, over-active mucus membranes.

Requirements for Vitamin A

0 to 6 months	375 RE
6 to 12 months	375 RE
Age 1 to 3 years	400 RE
Age 4 to 6 years	500 RE
Age 7 to 10 years	700 RE
Males 11 to 14 years	1,000 RE
Males 15 to 18 years	1,000 RE
Females 11 to 14 years	800 RE
Females 15 to18 years	800 RE

VITAMIN B COMPLEX

Function: B vitamins promote digestion, growth, and appetite. They maintain the health of nerves and thr brain. There are increased requirements for the B vitamins during nursing. B complex vitamins help prevent degenerative diseases, such as arthritis. They aid in protein metabolism and help prevent tooth decay, edema, and epileptic seizures.

Sources: wild rice, bran, sprouts, almonds, legumes, dark green leafy vegetables, raw fruit, whole grains.

Enemies: alcohol, caffeine, coffee, sugar, tobacco, oral contraceptives, excess starches, sleeping pills, estrogen, stress, sulfa drugs.

Deficiency Signs: beriberi, pellagra, digestive disorders, poor appetite, restless leg syndrome, tongue that is cracked, shiny, or purple, memory loss, confusion, canker sores, weight loss, nervous and glandular disorders, fatigue, depression, itchy/burning eyes, eczema, brittle nails, linked to birth defects.

Requirements for Thiamin

0 to 6 months	0.3 mg
6 to 12 months	0.4 mg
Age 1 to 3 years	0.7 mg
Age 4 to 6 years	0.9 mg
Age 7 to 10 years	1.0 mg
Males 11 to 14 years	1.3 mg
Males 15 to18 years	1.5 mg
Females 11 to 14 years	1.1 mg
Females 15 to 18 years	1.1 mg

Requirements for Riboflavin

0 to 6 months	0.4 mg
6 to 12 months	0.5 mg
Age 1 to 3 years	0.8 mg
Age 4 to 6 years	1.1 mg
Age 7 to 10 years	1.2 mg
Males 11 to 14 years	1.5 mg
Males 15 to 18 years	1.8 mg
Females 11 to 14 years	1.3 mg
Females 15 to 18 years	1.3 mg

Requirements for Niacin

0 to 6 months	5 mg
6 to 12 months	5 mg
Age 1 to 3 years	9 mg
Age 4 to 6 years	12 mg
Age 7 to 10 years	13 mg
Males 11 to 14 years	17 mg
Males 15 to 18 years	20 mg
Females 11 to 14 years	15 mg
Females 15 to 18 years	15 mg

VITAMIN C

Function: C is essential for healthy collagen, the "glue" that holds cells together. It is necessary for vital function of all organs and glands. Vitamin C protects against stress (physical and mental), toxic chemicals, and some poisons. C acts as a natural antibiotic and promotes healing. It aids in maintaining healthy sex organs and adrenal glands. Vitamin C assists in healthy tooth formation.

Sources: all raw fruits and vegetables, especially red bell peppers, tomatoes, citrus fruit, green leafy vegetables, sprouts.

Enemies: alcohol, antibiotics, aspirin, barbiturates, cooking heat, cortisone, high fevers, pain killers, stress, tobacco.

Deficiency Signs: bruises easily, scurvy, mouth/gum disease, fragile bones and joints, gastric ulcers, frequent cold and flu, cancer, anemia, adrenal malfunction, stiff joints, asthma, bronchitis.

Requirements for Vitamin C

0 to 6 months	30 mg
6 to 12 months	35 mg
Age 1 to 3 years	40 mg
Age 4 to 6 years	45 mg
Age 7 to 10 years	45 mg
Males 11 to 14 years	50 mg
Males 15 to 18 years	60 mg
Females 11 to 14 years	50 mg
Females 15 to 18 years	60 mg

VITAMIN D

Function: D is essential for utilization of calcium and other metals by the digestive tract. It is necessary for proper function of thyroid and other glands. Vitamin D assures proper formation of bones and teeth in children.

Sources: exposure of uncovered skin to the sun, fish-liver oils, raw milk, egg yolks, sprouted seeds, mushrooms.

Enemies: barbiturates, cortisone, mineral oil, sleeping pills, smog.

Deficiency Signs: bone disease, rickets, cataracts, calcium malabsorption, gum disease, hair loss, muscle weakness, tooth decay, retarded growth, osteoporosis.

Requirements for Vitamin D

0 to 6 months	7.5 mcg
6 to 12 months	10 mcg
Age 1 to 3 years	10 mcg
Age 4 to 6 years	10 mcg
Age 7 to 10 years	10 mcg
Males 11 to 14 years	10 mcg
Males 15 to 18 years	10 mcg
Females 11 to 14 years	10 mcg
Females 15 to 18 years	10 mcg

VITAMIN E

Function: E provides oxygen to tissues and cells. Vitamin E improves circulation. It prevents and reduces scar tissue. E retards aging, lessens menopausal disorders. It is essential for the health of reproductive organs. Vitamin E also serves as an anticoagulant.

Sources: raw and sprouted seeds and grains, legumes, eggs, dark green leafy vegetables, nuts.

Enemies: chlorine, heat, mineral oil, rancid fats and oils, oral contraceptives.

Deficiency Signs: cardiovascular and circulatory disorders, premature aging, hot flashes, female problems, impotence, nervous system imbalances, weakened immune system.

Requirements for Vitamin E

0 to 6 months	3 mg
6 to 12 months	4 mg
Age 1 to 3 years	6 mg
Age 4 to 6 years	7 mg
Age 7 to 10 years	7 mg
Males 11 to 14 years	10 mg
Males 15 to 18 years	10 mg
Females 11 to 14 years	8 mg
Females 15 to 18 years	8 mg

1 mg of natural vitamin E = 1 IU

VITAMIN K

Function: Vitamin K is vital for blood clotting and liver function. It also aids in vitality and longevity.

Sources: seeds, sprouts, raw milk, alfalfa, kelp.

Enemies: N/A

Deficiency Signs: hemorrhoids, bruising, hemorrhaging, delayed blood clotting, colon and liver disorders, MS, leg ulcers, diverticulitis, colitis, intestinal disorders.

Requirements for Vitamin K

0 to 6 months	5 mcg
6 to 12 months	10 mcg
Age 1 to 3 years	15 mcg
Age 4 to 6 years	20 mcg
Age 7 to 10 years	30 mcg
Males 11 to 14 years	45 mcg
Males 15 to 18 years	65 mcg
Females 11 to 14 years	45 mcg
Females 15 to 18 years	55 mcg

CALCIUM

Function: Calcium is vital for all muscle and body activities. It is needed for building and maintaining bones and for normal growth, heart action, and blood clotting. It is essential for normal pregnancy and lactation. Calcium must be present for magnesium to be utilized.

Sources: sesame seeds (more than milk), tahini, raw milk, dark green leafy vegetables, kelp, sea vegetables.

Enemies: aspirin, chocolate, mineral oil, oxalic acid, stress.

Deficiency Signs: muscle spasms, bone softening, insomnia, hypertension, menopause, colitis, rheumatism, rickets.

Requirements for Calcium

0 to 6 months	400 mg
6 to 12 months	600 mg
Age 1 to 3 years	800 mg
Age 4 to 6 years	800 mg
Age 7 to 10 years	800 mg
Males 11 to 14 years	1200 mg
Males 15 to 18 years	1200 mg
Females 11 to 14 years	1200 mg
Females 15 to 18 years	1200 mg

CHROMIUM

Function: Chromium is necessary for utilization of sugar. It is involved with activity of hormones and enzymes. Chromium aids in metabolism of cholesterol. It is identified as a glucose tolerance factor. Chromium helps regulate serum cholesterol.

Sources: whole grain cereals, Brewer's yeast, grain sprouts, mushrooms.

Enemies: refined carbohydrates, sugar.

Deficiency Signs: depressed growth rate, glucose intolerance in diabetics, hypoglycemia, fatigue, memory and muscle loss, weight problems, heart disorder.s

Requirements for Chromium

0 to 6 months	10 – 40 mcg
6 to 12 months	20 – 60 mcg
Age 1 to 3 years	20 – 80 mcg
Age 4 to 6 years	30 – 120 mcg
Age 7 to 10 years	50 – 200 mcg
Males 11 to 14 years	50 – 200 mcg
Males 15 to 18 years	50 – 200 mcg
Females 11 to 14 years	50 – 200 mcg
Females 15 to 18 years	50 – 200 mcg

IRON

Function: Iron is necessary for formation of red blood cells, which transport oxygen to all body cells. Quality hemoglobin provides resistance to disease and stress.

Sources: blackstrap molasses, raisins, prunes, nuts, seeds, whole grains, sea vegetables, sprouts, legumes.

Enemies: coffee, some food additives.

Deficiency Signs: headaches, listlessness and fatigue, irritability, heart palpitations during exertion, dizziness, reduced white blood cell count, impaired antibody production, anemia, pale color.

Requirements for Iron

0 to 6 months	6 mg
6 to 12 months	10 mg
Age 1 to 3 years	10 mg
Age 4 to 6 years	10 mg
Age 7 to 10 years	10 mg

Males 11 to 14 years	12 mg
Males 15 to 18 years	12 mg
Females 11 to 14 years	15 mg
Females 15 to 18 years	15 mg

MAGNESIUM

Function: Magnesium is essential for enzyme activity. It aids in the body's use of Vitamin B and E, fats and other minerals, especially calcium. Magnesium helps provide strong bones and muscle tone. It contributes to a healthy heart. Magnesium balances acid-alkaline condition of the body. It helps prevent build-up of cholesterol.

Sources: sesame, sunflower, and pumpkin seeds, almonds, whole grains, green leafy vegetables, sprouts, apples, peaches, lemons.

Enemies: alcohol, diuretics, processed foods, refined flour, sugar, excess protein.

Deficiency Signs: tremors, convulsions, muscle contractions, confusions, irritability, behavioral disturbances, heart disorders, insomnia, hypertension, menopause, rapid pulse, teeth grinding, hyperactivity, fatigue, fear, anxiety, memory loss, fear.

Requirements for Magnesium

0 to 6 months	40 mg
6 to 12 months	60 mg
Age 1 to 3 years	80 mg
Age 4 to 6 years	120 mg
Age 7 to 10 years	170 mg
Males 11 to 14 years	270 mg
Males 15 to 18 years	400 mg
Females 11 to 14 years	280 mg
Females 15 to 18 years	300 mg

ZINC

Function: Zinc assists in healing wounds and burns. It contributes to protein and carbohydrate metabolism as well as healthy reproductive organs. Zinc effects the transfer of carbon dioxide from the tissues to the lungs.

Sources: wheat germ and bran, seeds, nuts, soy products.

Enemies: alcohol, food processing, oral contraceptives, stress, excess calcium.

Deficiency Signs: impaired ability to heal, loss of appetite, impaired night vision, impairment of taste and smell, retarded growth, impotence, infertility, colds and flu, fatigue, hair loss, skin lesions, acne, skeletal abnormalities.

Requirements for Zinc

0 to 6 months	5 mg
6 to 12 months	5 mg
Age 1 to 3 years	10 mg
Age 4 to 6 years	10 mg
Age 7 to 10 years	10 mg
Males 11 to 14 years	15 mg
Males 15 to 18 years	15 mg
Females 11 to 14 years	12 mg
Females 15 to 18 years	12 mg

MEDIAN HEIGHTS, WEIGHTS AND SUGGESTED CALORIC INTAKES BY AGE:

Age	**Weight**	**Height**	**Calories**
0 to 6 months	13 lb.	24 in.	650
6 to 12 months	20 lb.	28 in.	850
Age 1 to 3 years	29 lb.	35 in.	1300

Age	Weight	Height	Calories
Age 4 to 6 years	44 lb.	44 in.	1800
Age 7 to 10 years	62 lb.	52 in.	2000
Males 11 to 14 years	99 lb.	62 in.	2500
Males 15 to 18 years	145 lb.	69 in.	3000
Females 11 to 14 years	101 lb.	62 in.	2200
Females 15 to 18 years	120 lb.	64 in.	2200

These Recommended Dietary Allowances and median heights, weights, and suggested caloric intakes are from the Food and Nutrition Board, National Academy of Sciences — National Research Council, revised in 1989.

CHAPTER EIGHT

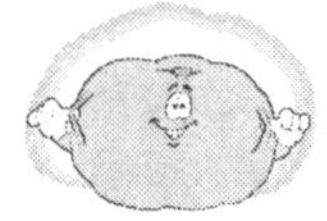

A physically fit child becomes a physically fit adult.

Building Physical Fitness

In order to be healthy, a child must be physically fit. In today's society of TV watching and minimal exercise, our children are often not physically fit. TV not only prevents children from getting the exercise they need, it also plays continuous ads for nutritionally void snacks as well as modeling rebellion as a desirable activity. Regular television viewing promotes a mindless state close to a coma. Watching TV encourages a viewer mentality instead of participatory action. I encourage you to eliminate or greatly limit TV viewing. Don't let the television become the family substitute for parenting, exercise, and childhood role models.

To be physically fit, the lungs and heart must be strong. Joints and muscles must be flexible and the muscles must also be strong to increase physical endurance. Balanced weight is also critical. Obesity is often caused by the lack of exercise more than just merely overeating, although that can also be a contributor. In actuality, the primary contributor to weight problems is exercise, followed by malnutrition. Eating the wrong food and not enough of the right foods, as well as not digesting or assimilating foods, can easily cause obesity in children as well as adults.[1]

The more the heart, lungs, and blood work together, the healthier the body. Regular exercise, if aerobic, forces the heart and lungs to work together while pulling in extra oxygen for the blood. All muscles need oxygen to function. Oxygen is important in building the immune system and creating an environment to fight free radicals, which are a precursor of cancer.

Flexibility is marked by how easily joints and muscles move. The elbow, knee, back, and hip all have a range of motion. A child who can freely move each of these joints, is considered flexible. Flexible joints are less prone to accidents. Inactivity causes stiff joints and, often, lower back pain. Stretching is one of the best ways to keep muscles and joints flexible. Muscle strength is the ability to exert force over a period of time. Resistance exercise (exercising "against" something) builds muscle strength.

With the increase of health problems such as obesity and osteoporosis, it is critical to lay down a foundation of exercise with children early. Osteoporosis often occurs due to a lack of density in the bones. Density comes from weight-bearing exercise and nutrition. Weight-bearing exercise includes running, walking, and tennis. Sports such as swimming do not add weight and therefore do not prevent osteoporosis. Getting your children walking early, especially through family walks, increases the fitness, physical health, and emotional well being of your child. Take the time to go for a walk with your child. You need that exercise, too!

---

[1] Leo Galland and Dian Dincin Buchman, *Superimmunity for Kids* (New York: Copestone Press, Inc., 1988), 196.

One of the most overlooked treatments for hyperactivity is exercise. Although hyper children seem to have too much energy, they usually have poor coordination and motor skills.[2] Helping your child to develop combined coordination between arm, head, and leg, through regular, planned exercise, can be very helpful. Other exercises to help with hyperactivity include trampoline jumping, dancing, gymnastics, and crawling on all fours.

As you work on the physical fitness of your child, it is important to know what he/she is capable of doing at the various age levels. As you work within the physical abilities with emotional and nutritional encouragement, you will help promote overall fitness and wellness in your child. The following tips are to help you know what children are able to do at different ages. Remember, some children will vary in development somewhat. However, as they grow older, the variation should be less.

ACTIVITIES AT VARIOUS AGES AND THE RELATED DEVELOPMENT

0 TO 3 MONTHS

Development

First year development follows three rules of thumb: (1) control of movement proceeds from the head downward, (2) motor control of limbs develops down the limbs (arms before wrists before fingers), (3) movements progress from general to specific (patting an object to reaching to grasping).[3]

---

[2] Marcea Weber, *Encyclopedia of Natural Health and Healing for Children* (Roccklin, CA: Prima Publishing, 1992), 175.

[3] Mike Samuels and Nancy Samuels, *The Well Baby Book* (New York: Simon & Schuster, 1991), 155.

As a newborn, a baby can move his/her head from right to left to prevent suffocating. By about one month they have started to lift their heads off of a flat surface. Within a few weeks a newborn's movements become less jerky and more smooth. Over the first few months, babies develop more head control. By about the third month, they can stretch their arms out and actually raise their heads and chests. During this time, head control will also increase while they are in a sitting position. Since a baby's head is four times bigger in proportion to its body (in comparison to an adult), gaining head control requires major effort.

Activity Tips

To promote development use a variety of shapes, sounds, and textures. Keep items small enough for the child to grasp, yet big enough to keep out of the mouth. Hold toys away from the child to encourage stretching and eventually grasping. Arouse the baby's interest with the use of rattles or other gentle noisemakers. Hang objects from a bar over the crib. When changing diapers, gently push and pull your child's arms and legs to encourage flexibility.

3 TO 6 MONTHS

Development

Approximately during this phase (remember each child is different), a child will begin to turn over from stomach to back and in reverse motion. The first time a baby does this, it may be startling or even frightening. But the child quickly learns to enjoy the process and his/her increasing control. Rolling over means a baby has " mobility." Watch out, your life will never be the same. At about the same time, a baby begins to sit without support. This accomplishment allows a child to play with both hands. What fun!

Activity Tips

At this age, a child is interested in reaching, grasping and turning over. Pat-a-cake can become a favorite activity. Playpens, although convenient, should be used minimally. A "jumper chair" hung in a doorway is a great use of extra energy. Do not use for extended periods of time, as it will lead to fatigue (for the child, not you).

To help develop head control, place the baby in a carrier or pack, as soon as the neck and head are sufficiently well developed. Place the infant on its stomach to encourage the use of head and neck muscles. When the baby is on his back, gently pull him to a sitting position to help him develop his upper body muscles.

To help develop rolling abilities, place a baby on its stomach frequently. You can also place the baby on a tilted surface (i.e., your bed, with your hand pushing down to cause a decline). This height variation gently encourages the child to roll over. In addition, placing something visually interesting near the baby's head can encourage the child to reach for it and thereby turn over.

6 TO 9 MONTHS

Development

During this age a child begins the process of learning to crawl. Crawling, the reciprocal use of arm to arm and leg to leg, has been associated with the ability to read at a later age. Strongly encourage your child to crawl and not just skip on to walking. At about 6 months, a baby can stand and support its own body weight. They will also begin to flex their knees while standing. At some point during this phase, they will begin to pull themselves up on anything they can find. Be careful they don't topple heavy items over on themselves.

Activity Tips

It's tub time. At this time, children will love to take a bath and it is great exercise for them. You will also want to childproof your house by now. Crawling children can find anything and move with unbelievable speed. Turn your head for a second and they're off!

Placing your hands at the bottom of your child's feet while he/she is are on the floor allows the child to "push off". This introduces the baby to the crawling sensation. To encourage crawling, place toys just out of reach of the baby. Calling to a baby, while out of reach to him, will also encourage crawling.

9 TO 12 MONTHS

Development

Walking can begin from now through the first months after age 1. Watch out for sharp-edged tables or other obstacles that can get in the way. Walkers can be helpful in the beginning to help strengthen legs. Do not use for too long, let the child move on his own.

Activity Tips

Be sure to keep an eagle eye out for your totally mobile child. They can, and will, move at the speed of light. At this age they will enjoy pushing and pulling type toys. Even though their attention span is still short, they will enjoy any activity with mom and dad. Take time to play with your child. Play is essential exercise to them.

AGE 1 TO 2

Development

At this age, children can be crawling, walking, or running. Allow your child to fall and get back up without your help. This builds strength and confidence. Don't build fear by fussing over each fall.

Activity Tips

Wagons and carts (push-pull toys), beach balls and soft foam toys can be fun for children at this age. Batting large balloons helps develop eye/hand coordination. Giving piggy back rides or gently roughhousing can be enjoyed by you and your child.

AGE 2

Development

Between 2 and 3, it is estimated that a child has grown to half of his/her adult height. Let your child run, jump, and explore. Look for playgrounds that have more than the standard slides and swings. Climbing is especially good for growing muscles. They should be able to balance on one foot for one second. Encourage them to jump in place and begin to jump with both feet together.

Activity Tips

Expose your child to outdoor play areas that stimulate large motor skills. Jungle gyms, swings, and slides are great for encouraging fitness. Let the child play with push-pull toys. Encourage outdoor activity as well as indoor.

AGE 3 TO 5

Development

Pedaling a tricycle or bike is a feat children are most proud of. They can begin to skip rope, hop on one foot, and learn to catch and throw. Children will enjoy inventing their own games and playing with other children. Children need daily, outdoor activity.

At the age of 4 or 5, children should be able to run smoothly, catch a ball to their chests and walk on a 2" or 3" beam, using foot-over-foot alternating steps. As they move into the next year, they should be able to jump, catch a ball using hands to grasp, kick a rolled ball, and punt a ball. Dribbling a ball with one hand and riding a 2-wheel bike without training wheels are skills that usually come during the fifth year.

Activity Tips

Encourage your child to try ladders, ropes, balance beams, see-saws, balls, and bikes. Let them try to develop in areas of strength and weakness. Playhouses can help them with imagination as well as drama, which uses all of the large muscles. Playing tag, hide and seek, and other small group games can help develop large motor skills and interaction with others.

AGE 6 TO 7

Development

At this age, boys and girls are physiologically equal. Their organs and bones are immature and consequently susceptible to injury. It is usually recommended to avoid high-impact sports such as football, hockey, and lacrosse until the child is more fully developed.

It is at this age that your child may become interested in organized sports. If you introduce your child to organized sports, be sure to stress the fun component and not just the competition. Allow them to have a good time.

Both boys and girls are still flexible, yet stretching exercises are probably some of the most important for this age. Most children this age are not interested in resistance exercise, which bears minimal benefits at this age. Be sure to make exercise fun. During the sixth year, children can learn to gallop skillfully, slide on two feet (as on ice), skip, and hop on one foot.

Activity Tips

Encourage activity instead of television viewing. Children usually are not yet aware of how they are different in physical development compared to other children their age. Encourage children to try new activities. Take time to help them learn how to accomplish various physical skills. Walking continues to be an excellent activity.

AGE 8 TO 10

Development

Kids this age begin to be aware of their physical abilities. This can lead to shame or pride. Kids who are not physically well developed can begin to feel inadequate and drop out of sports. It is estimated that 80% to 90% of all children drop out of organized sports by the age of 15 or 16.[4]

During this age, children can throw, dribble a soccer ball with their feet, and strike a moving object such as a baseball. Carefully monitor the sports your child becomes involved in to minimize developing any negative attitudes. Keep as many activities as possible non-competitive.

Girls and boys are still similar to each other in physical development at this stage. Bone-growth plates are open and this age group is still vulnerable to injury, so avoid high-impact sports. Keep them stretching, as many kids this age are beginning to loose flexibility.

Activity Tips

Schedule 20 minutes of aerobic exercise three days each week. Make it fun by enrolling your child in a community club or class. If you are involved in regular exercise (I'm sure you are, right?), include your child in your activities. Skiing, swimming, running, or bike riding can be great adult/child activities. Emotional bonding and "together time" is also provided in adult/child exercise.

---

[4] Arnold Schwarzenegger, *Arnold's Fitness for Kids* (New York: Doubleday, 1993), 23.

Supplement this planned exercise and school exercise with games and exercise at home. Don't assume your child is getting all of his or her needed exercise at school. Many kids just stand and talk during recess periods. If you are homeschooling, take the time for planned exercise as part of your curriculum. When exercising in any way, be sure children drink lots of water as their bodies get hotter than adults.

TEENS

Unless your teen has developed athletic skills and is actively involved in sports, chances are your teen is getting no exercise. Most teens have become observers in life in more ways than one. They are often embarrassed at their bodies and all of their physical changes. They often avoid physical activity as it promotes a sense of inadequacy. If this tendency is not checked and corrected during this phase, this attitude will probably roll right into adulthood.

If you have not taken the time prior to this to encourage and role model physical activity, you have a challenge ahead of you. You will need to discuss the situation with your teen. They will need to fully participate in the decision process to begin more exercising. Finding an activity they can enjoy may take time and creativity.

Eliminating television can be of help. Television strongly promotes non-activity. Taking the time to join your teen in exercise can encourage one-on-one time which teens cherish, even if they don't say so. Never underestimate the value of your time with a teen. The pressures and choices confronting our teens today are way beyond the choices we faced as teens. Having an outlet through physical exercise and adult companionship can help a teen deal with these stress-filled years. Learning to make wise choices in regard to their physical bodies can be a struggle for most teens.

Keeping children physically fit through regular exercise can help set a routine in place that becomes invaluable as they reach adulthood. Many adults have trouble establishing regular exercise because of childhood neglect of physical development. It is hard to start swimming, jumping rope, skiing, cycling, etc., as an adult if you never experienced it as a child. Expose your child to many different physical activities with as much variety as possible. Be assured, one of those will pique their interest and you will have helped establish a lifelong habit of physical opportunity and fitness.

CHAPTER NINE

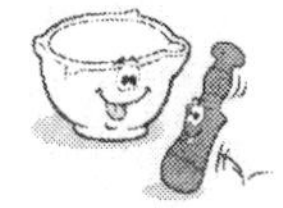

Knowing how to handle common childhood ailments provides a parent confidence and direction.

Handling Common Childhood Ailments

As parents we want to do the best for our children. As they encounter various childhood ailments, knowing how to deal with them provides a parent confidence and direction. We will address several common ailments. We will give a general overview and suggestions for handling the problem. These suggestions are not meant as prescriptions or to replace the advice of your health care provider. For more detail on the covered topics and for ailments not covered in this book, please check out the references contained in Appendix A.

Secondly, this chapter will help you build a natural home health kit. This kit can also be used for travel and camping. Having the right natural remedies can save a lot of grief and discomfort for your child when a problem arises.

Finally, you will find the last section of this chapter helps you find a holistic health care provider. The suggestions will help you know how to interview a practitioner and how to find people to interview.

COMMON GUIDE TO SYMPTOMS

In their book, *Smart Medicine for a Healthier Child* (Garden City Park, NY: Avery Publishing Group, 1994), Janet Zand, Rachel Walton, and Bob Rountree, provide an excellent reference for common childhood symptoms. I highly recommend this book for its detailed discussion and practical solutions to all childhood ailments.

The following chart is a summary of their guide, my experience, and research of numerous other books.

Symptom	**Possible Causes**
Abdominal Pain	Appendicitis, colic, constipation, diarrhea, emotional upset, food allergies, intestinal obstruction, motion sickness, urinary tract infection
Anal Itching	Parasites, yeast infection
Increased Appetite	Diabetes, overexertion, thyroid disorders
Loss of Appetite	Appendicitis, cancer, constipation, mumps, teething, thrush
Bedwetting	Common cold, diabetes, emotional upset, allergies, urinary tract infection
Painful Bowel Movement	Colitis, constipation, rectal fissure
Difficulty Breathing	Allergies, asthma, croup, inhaled foreign body, rheumatic fever, shock, tetanus
Rapid Breathing	Asthma, croup, pneumonia, shock

Symptom	Possible Causes
Cold Sweat	Shock
Cough	Allergies, asthma, bronchitis, common cold, croup, emotional upset, viral or bacterial infection
Diarrhea	Food poisoning, viral or bacterial infection
Earache	Allergies, common cold, ear infection, rapid air pressure changes
Difficulty Eating	Cancer, canker sores, allergies, mononucleosis, mumps, sore throat, teething, thrush
Eye Inflammation	Allergies, common cold, environmental toxins, onset of measles, sty
Fatigue	Anemia, cancer, diabetes, depression, allergies, poor digestion
Head Itching	Eczema, environmental toxins, lice, psoriasis
Headache	Allergies, chickenpox, common cold, concussion, emotional upset, mononucleosis, motion sickness, mumps, stress, visual problems
Irritability	Allergies, asthma, colic, diabetes, emotional upset, hyperactivity, immunization reaction, meningitis, teething

Symptom	Possible Causes
Aching Joints	German measles, juvenile rheumatoid arthritis, nutritional deficiencies (i.e., calcium)
Swollen Lymph Nodes	Bacterial or viral infection, dermatitis, herpes virus, lice
Mouth Sores	Allergies, canker sores, onset of measles, thrush
Runny Nose	Allergies, bronchitis, common cold, measles, sinusitis
Seizure	Epilepsy, fever, head injury, immunization reaction
Skin Rash	Acne, allergies, athlete's foot, boils, chickenpox, cradle cap, immunization reaction, prickly heat, sunburn, warts
Excessive Thirst	Dehydration, diabetes
Frequent Urination	Diabetes, excessive caffeine, urinary tract infection
Painful Urination	Urinary tract infection, yeast infection
Dark Urine	Dehydration, hepatitis, urinary tract infection
Vaginal Itching	Allergic reaction, yeast infection
Vomiting	Allergic reaction, appendicitis, emotional upset, food poisoning, meningitis, motion sickness, overeating, shock
Weight Loss	Cancer, diabetes, eating disorder, depression

The following list of ailments includes the most common ailments children might experience. We will briefly cover fevers, headaches, abdominal pains, coughs, runny noses, earaches, skin problems, asthma and allergies, hyperactivity and ADD, constipation and diarrhea, and obesity.

Fevers

Your child feels hot. You take his/her temperature and find it is over 100 degrees. You panic and immediately telephone your pediatrician. The most common response is to give the child an aspirin and take him/her to the doctor's office.

Let's take another approach. Robert Mendelsohn, M.D. says " …the presence of fever, by itself, does not mean that he (a doctor) should do anything at all. Unless there are additional symptoms, …your doctor should tell you there is nothing to worry about and send you and your child home."[1] Be sure to check with your doctor regarding fevers in newborn babies.

The "normal" temperature of 98.6 degrees Fahrenheit is a statistical average. Therefore, a child's temperature can vary and still be normal for him. Temperatures can vary throughout the day, after a heavy meal or when taking medication.

Fever temperatures can also vary based on where they are taken. Rectal temperatures usually register higher than oral temperatures. Underarm temperatures usually register lower. Knowing this, the underarm approach is usually easier and less traumatic for all involved.

With babies or infants, (children under six months of age) check to see if they are overdressed. Many parents overdress a child wanting to be "good parents." A simple rule is to dress your baby the same way you need to dress for the climate.

---

[1] Robert Mendelsohn, *How to Raise a Healthy Child... In Spite of Your Doctor* (New York: Ballantine Books, 1984), 74.

Most fevers are caused by viral and bacterial infections, which the child's own defense mechanisms will overcome, if given a chance. A common cold can elevate temperatures all the way to 105 degrees. The primary risk is dehydration.[2] Make sure your child is getting enough fluids.

Research shows no link between disease severity and the height of a child's temperature.[3] Knowing the temperature does not inform you of how sick your child is. Some serious diseases produce no elevated temperature at all.

Fevers actually indicate the body is doing its work. When an infection develops, white cell activity increases. This increased activity raises body temperature. Hence the fever. An elevated temperature simply means the healing process is working. Attempting to lower the fever can be counterproductive. Mendelsohn and other natural health care providers recommend letting the fever run its course, unless other more serious symptoms are present. Interfering with a fever often interrupts the healing process.

Fevers that are serious are usually fairly obvious. They usually stem from poisoning, exposure to toxic substances, or heat stroke. If you suspect your child has swallowed poison, call your poison center immediately. If your child lapses into unconsciousness and has a fever, take the child to the emergency room promptly. This combination of symptoms can be extremely serious.

GENERAL RECOMMENDATIONS

- ••• Drink lots of fluids.
- ••• Give your child an echinacea and goldenseal combination formula.

---

[2] Mendelsohn, *How to Raise a Healthy Child... In Spite of Your Doctor*, 7.

[3] Ibid, 78.

- ••• Encourage your child to lie down and rest. Watch him and do not let him become chilled.
- ••• Fever-reducing herbal teas may help naturally lower the temperature.
- ••• Avoid sponging or bathing with cold water or rubbing alcohol. The cold temperatures cause the blood vessels to constrict, making the body heat more difficult to release.
- ••• Vitamin C can be helpful in treating fevers from minor infections.
- ••• Feed your child as little as possible during the first 24 hours of a fever. This type of temporary fasting helps stimulate the immune system.
- ••• It is common for constipation to occur during fevers. This added toxicity in the body may even stimulate the fever. A gentle cleanse of the bowels after a fever can be helpful.
- ••• Check with your health care provider for homeopathic, herbal, and other nutritional support.

Headaches

Almost any abnormal physical, emotional, mental, or spiritual condition in a child can promote a headache. The most common source for headaches in children is viral or bacterial infection in the body. The next most frequent source is emotional stress. Headaches are so common that current statistics say that 20% of school age children complain of headaches.[4]

Headaches can be separated into categories: migraine and other types. Migraines are rare in children, unless there is a family history. Most other types of headaches are often allergy

[4] Weber, *Encyclopedia of Natural Health and Healing for Children*, 167.

related as in the case of sinus headaches and tension headaches. Sinus headaches are often accompanied with nasal congestion or postnasal drip and tend to worsen with damp weather. Chronic sinus headaches are usually caused by allergy to molds in the air or to foods or both.[5]

If the headache is due to mold allergies, eliminating foods containing mold (or its cousin, yeast) can be helpful. This includes foods such as sugar, bread, cheese, prepared foods, fermented foods, yeast, and apple cider. Headaches from food sensitivities or allergies indicate a weak liver and/or digestive system.

Tension headaches can be caused by eye strain, indicating a need for glasses. They can also be caused by poor posture, lack of neck movement, and spinal disorientation.

Keeping a child fed with nutritious foods, exposed to fresh air, and well exercised while omitting foods high in sugar, saturated fat, and spices will be an excellent preventer of many headaches.

GENERAL RECOMMENDATIONS

- Supplementing with acidophilus can help decrease the growth of yeast in the intestine.
- Taking Kyolic garlic supplements can help enhance the immune system's yeast killing abilities.
- If the child is over the age of 8 to 10, hee/she may often benefit from taking digestive supplements to strengthen the digestive system. Additionally, a mild liver cleanse may be helpful in older children.
- Resting in a darkened room with a cool cloth on the forehead can be helpful.

[5] Galland and Buchman, *Superimmunity for Kids*, 209.

- ••• A massage or bath with a few drops of the essential oil of Lavender or Rosemary may help.
- ••• An elimination diet, under a health care provider's supervision, can help identify food allergies. Omitting these foods can help minimize or eliminate allergy-related headaches.
- ••• Supplementing a child's diet with EFA (Essential Fatty Acids) such as fish oils or flaxseed oil can help thin the blood and block the cycle that promotes chronic headaches.
- ••• Many herbal and nutritional remedies are available with help from a natural health care provider.

Abdominal Pains

"Tummy aches" can vary in location and cause. They can be caused by allergies, improper intestinal flora, a toxic digestive system (undigested food), or by overeating or eating too fast. One of the most frequent causes of abdominal pain is (milk) intolerances. Children who were not nursed often do not have the right balance of stomach bacteria for good digestion.

Offering a child an antacid can compound the problem. If the "tummy ache" is not in the stomach, the antacid will be of no help. If the ache really is from excess acid, an antacid will remove the stomach's acid, causing the stomach to produce more and a repetitive cycle to occurs.

If a child's abdominal pain is accompanied by vomiting or diarrhea, or headaches for more than 24 hours, talk to your health care provider. This abdominal pain could be an indicator of appendicitis.

GENERAL RECOMMENDATIONS

- ••• Encourage your child to go to the bathroom and have a bowel movement.

- ••• Herbal teas, such as peppermint (helps digestion) or chamomile (helps relax), can be soothing and help reduce abdominal pain.
- ••• Omit common allergenic foods, such as eggs, dairy products, and processed food using white flour and sugar.
- ••• Review your child's day to determine if some emotional upset could be the culprit.

Coughs, Runny Noses and Colds

Since it takes time for a child's immune system to become strong, colds, coughs, and runny noses may be frequent. These symptoms can also be an indicator of allergies and environmental toxins.

Mucus membranes are being effected by these symptoms. Excessive mucus production in the throat or sinus cavities irritates the main bronchi, causing coughing. This overproduction of mucus can stem from infection, over-tiredness, emotional trauma, or mucus-producing foods (i.e., dairy products).

A cough occurs when the trachea or windpipe becomes infected. To fight infection, the throat produces a thicker mucus called phlegm. The child coughs in order to eliminate phlegm.

Nursed infants have fewer colds than older children. This is probably due to immunity passed along in breast milk. Babies under age 1, with cold symptoms, may have more nasal congestion, a fever, and mild diarrhea. Colds in 1 to 2-year-olds come quickly and usually are short lived. As a child reaches the age of 3 or 4, colds are more like adult colds.

GENERAL RECOMMENDATIONS

- ••• Be sure the child consumes extra fluids to prevent dehydration. Fluids also help break up the congestion from excess mucus.

- Eliminate mucus causing foods, such as milk and dairy products, wheat and bread products. This would not include breast milk.
- Vaporizers can help add moisture to the air and help relax children. A cool mist vaporizer is safer than hot mist. A hot shower can help older children.
- Ensure your child is getting plenty of rest so that the body can begin the process of healing itself.
- The use of a baby syringe for babies who can't nurse due to stuffy noses can be helpful.
- Gentle massage of the chest or mild exercise can help loosen and remove mucus.
- Caster oil packs applied to the chest, covered with a couple of layers of towels and warmed by a hot water bottle can also help.
- Many herbal, homeopathic remedies are available for more specific symptoms.

Earaches

Earaches are one of the most common childhood complaints. Paul Berner in the November/December 1991 issue of the East-West Journal said, "Minor ear infections are the most common medical problem in children under six years of age in the U.S. — about one out of ten will have at least one infection annually."

Of these complaints, the most common is otitis media, or inflammation of the middle ear, which is usually caused by a viral infection with a secondary bacterial infection. The most common causes of earaches are allergies (i.e., dairy, wheat, etc.) and inhalants (i.e., dust, animal hair, and pollen). These contributors cause swollen tissues that prevent secretion drainage through the Eustachian tube. This becomes a breeding ground for bacteria. The Eustachian tube can also become blocked with impacted ear wax and water (i.e., swimming).

Earaches can also be impacted by a foreign object; overtiredness; fatty, greasy, oily, or spicy foods; over-excitement; sudden weather changes; atmospheric changes (i.e., plane or elevator), and emotional traumas.

Some professionals will inform parents that not treating an earache can lead to deafness. Dr. Robert Mendelsohn in his book "*How to Raise a Healthy Child... in Spite of Your Doctor*" says, "Many of my patients, perhaps the majority, failed to take their antibiotics (for earaches) …or get the prescription filled at all. What disturbed me more than (this) noncompliance was the realization that my noncompliant patients recovered from their infections as rapidly as those who complied, and not one of them ever went deaf."[6] Dr. Mendelsohn also does not recommend antibiotics, decongestants, antihistamines, or tympanostomies (plastic tubes) for patients with earaches.

In a Netherlands study of 171 children (double-blind study) studied by Dr. Mendelsohn, the result showed: "Half were treated with antibiotics, and the other half were not. There was no significant difference in the clinical course of the disease — pain, temperature, discharge from the ear, or change in the appearance of the ear drum or hearing levels — between those treated without antibiotics and those who received them."[7]

GENERAL RECOMMENDATIONS

- Relieve pain with a heating pad, a couple of drops of heated olive or garlic oil (not hot) inserted into the ear canal. A small cotton ball in the ear can keep the oil from dripping out. Repeat twice a day for no more than four days. (Discontinue if any side effects appear.)
- Don't use any instrument to forcibly remove wax.

[6] Mendelsohn, 145 – 6.

[7] Ibid, 147.

- ••• Question your health care provider's antibiotic prescription. Seek other options.
- ••• Check your child for food allergies or inhalants that could be causing chronic infections. Remove violators.
- ••• If your child does take antibiotics, follow their use with a sequence of live acidophilus to restore normal intestinal bacteria.
- ••• Temporarily remove all sugar (including juice and fruit) and dairy from your child's diet. When the earache leaves, slowly reintroduce these foods and see which ones he/she tolerates or reacts to.
- ••• Supplement your child's diet with EFA (essential fatty acids) in the form of flaxseed oil (1 to 2 teaspoons/day) or walnut oil (2 to 4 teaspoons/day).
- ••• Marcea Weber in her book *Encyclopedia of Natural Health and Healing for Children* recommends: peel and grate an onion. Squeeze out the juice. Warm the juice and apply 2 – 3 drops in the ear with an eye dropper or cotton wool. Works immediately.[8]
- ••• Have children 4 years and older gargle with 2 teaspoons sea salt and 2 teaspoons lemon juice added to 1 cup warm boiled water three times a day.
- ••• Have child drink plenty of water and use a vaporizer.

Skin Problems

Skin problems can show in the form of a rash. A rash can be flat, raised or blistered; red, pink, purple, or brown in color; moist and weepy, or dry and scaly; it may itch or it may not. Skin imbalances can cause diaper rash, eczema, acne, heat rash, and allergic rash reactions.

---

[8] Weber, 149.

Observe as much as you can about the skin reaction. For example, notice where the skin reaction occurs, its frequency, how it spreads, and any other symptoms. Be sure to note the prior activities of your child and any environmental factors (i.e., temperature, household toxins, potential allergens).

The most important rule in treating skin problems is cleanliness. Keep the affected area as clean as possible. The following lists possible rashes, descriptions, and possible solutions for many rashes.[9] For a more detailed review, see Janet Zand, Rachel Walton and Bob Rountree's book *Smart Medicine for a Healthier Child.*

Type of Rash	**Description**
Athlete's Foot	Clusters of tiny blisters and scaly sores between the toes. It usually itches and burns.

GENERAL RECOMMENDATIONS

- ••• Apply Tea-Tree oil directly to the affected area.
- ••• Rub a cider vinegar-soaked cloth between toes to remove scales.
- ••• Apply aloe vera gel to soothe itch.
- ••• Keep child's feet dry and clean.

Chickenpox	A flat, reddish rash that turns into batches of blisters and pimples. This itchy rash usually starts on the trunk and moves out the extremities, with few on the neck and head.

GENERAL RECOMMENDATIONS

- ••• Avoid the use of aspirin.
- ••• Calamine lotion or cold witch hazel applied to

[9] Zand, Walton, and Rountree, *Smart Medicine for a Healthier Child*, 370.

blisters may help relieve itching. Trim child's fingernails to minimize deep scratching.

- ••• Bathe in tepid water with added cornstarch or arrowroot.

Type of Rash	Description
Cradle Cap	Infants between 2 and 12 weeks can get thick, yellowish, crusty patches on the scalp, face, ears, or groin area. It is usuallly not itchy.

GENERAL RECOMMENDATIONS

- ••• Avoid too much shampooing and strong shampoos.
- ••• Breast-feeding moms should avoid refined sugar and saturated animal fats.
- ••• Increase intake of EFAs (essential fatty acids) in the form of salmon or flaxseed oil.
- ••• Rub affected area with calendula lotion and vitamin E oil, alternately.

Diaper Rash	Diaper rash, a red bottom area, can be caused by wetness, acidic urine (diet or hot weather), and acidic stool (caused by poor digestion). Allergies (food or chemical), teething, and illness can cause diaper rash.

GENERAL RECOMMENDATIONS

- ••• Use cloth or natural disposable diapers (see Appendix A). Change frequently. Avoid plastic pants.
- ••• Use loose, not tight clothing.
- ••• Avoid talc/most baby powders, they irritate wet skin.
- ••• Nursing mothers should avoid allergenic foods.
- ••• Avoid harsh laundry soaps.
- ••• Calendula gel or lotion can be soothing.

Type of Rash	Description
Eczema	Eczema is the most common symptom of allergies. It may be itchy, dry, wet, or a combination of all three. Nursed babies rarely develop eczema. Itching eczema is often caused by trapped poisons and toxins; dry eczema by poor digestion and mucus build up; wet eczema by poor digestion.

GENERAL RECOMMENDATIONS

- ••• Avoid allergenic foods in child and nursing mom.
- ••• Check for sensitivity of laundry products.
- ••• Apply olive oil, vitamin E oil, aloe vera gel, or calendula cream before bedtime twice a week.
- ••• Take oat baths (3 cups oatmeal tied in muslin bag added to bath water).
- ••• Vitamins C, E, and primrose oil can be helpful supplements.

Heat Rash	(Also known as prickly heat) is often caused by overdressing. It may appear as small, raised red lesions with tiny blisters at the center. May itch/sting.

GENERAL RECOMMENDATIONS

- ••• Apply calamine lotion or aloe vera gel. Bathe in cornstarch or oat baths.
- ••• Avoid refined sugar and high fat foods.

Hives	Hives are usually a food or drug allergenic reaction. The skin may swell and be itchy. Welts may be white-centered and ooze fluids.

GENERAL RECOMMENDATIONS

- ••• Eliminate allergenic source.
- ••• Apply calamine lotion or give cornstarch or oat baths.

Type of Rash	Description
Measles	Most common between the ages of 1 and 5. The incubation period is usually 10 to 14 days. The rash usually starts around the ears and hairline and spreads to the rest of the body over 3 to 4 days. It usually starts red and fades to a purple-red over a week.

GENERAL RECOMMENDATIONS

- ••• Ensure child is getting plenty of rest and fluids.
- ••• Use eyebright teas or diluted tinctures to bathe the eyes.
- ••• Provide plenty of fluids to prevent dehydration and promote healing.
- ••• Supplemental vitamins A, C, and zinc can be helpful.

Ringworm	A fungal infection that appears in circular patches of rough skin about the size of a nickel. Considered highly contagious.

GENERAL RECOMMENDATIONS

- ••• Apply Tea-Tree oil directly to the infected areas.
- ••• Provide a vegetable-rich diet for added nutrients.
- ••• Echinacea, goldenseal, and burdock herbal combinations can help.
- ••• Wash child's clothing after each wearing. Do not allow sharing of clothing, combs/brushes, socks or, bedding.

Asthma and Allergies

Approximately 10% of all school age children have wheezing and other asthma symptoms, and it is on the increase.[10] Frequent respiratory problems, emotional fears, and chronic mucus typify asthma sufferers. A rigid, expanded chest often occurs.

Asthma can be triggered by allergies (i.e., food, air-borne allergies, and inhalants), cigarette smoke, cold or dry air, infections, and stress.

The drugs used to treat asthma (inhalers containing beta-2-agonists) can contribute to asthma deaths over the long term.[11] These treatments may seem to help in the short term, but do seem to weaken the body over extended use.

GENERAL RECOMMENDATIONS

- Increase their intake of EFAs, especially flaxseed oil.
- Omit mucus-forming foods, such as dairy, wheat, citrus, eggs, and nuts.
- Drink lots of fluids.
- Alfalfa tablets or tea can soothe congestion.
- Avoid sulfites (used in commercial dried fruits, some vinegars, pickles, jams, beers, and some salad bars) and food additives.
- Supplements of magnesium, vitamins A, B6, B12, C, and licorice root can be helpful.

Hyperactivity and ADD

The medical term for hyperactivity is ADD (attention deficit disorder) or ADHD (attention deficit hyperactive disorder). Symptoms can include poor motor skills, memory problems, learning disorders (although child is usually average to above

---

[10] Weber, *Encyclopedia of Natural Health and Healing for Children*, 89.

[11] Ibid, 90.

average in intelligence), mood swings (may be aggressive), and poor concentration. Often people will believe these problems stem from "bad parenting."

One of the most common contributors to hyperactivity is food allergies. Dr. Ben Feingold (see Appendix A for more information) is a pioneer in the link of the impact of foods and chemicals on children's behavior (and adult's, too). Boys are ten times more likely to exhibit hyperactivity than girls.[12]

Drug therapy, such as Ritalin, has many side effects, such as insomnia, decreased appetite, weight loss, irritability, stomach aches, nausea, depression, and increased risk of cancer.

GENERAL RECOMMENDATIONS

- Check out allergies (food and chemical). Try a rotation or elimination diet under the supervision of your health care provider.
- Seek more information on the Feingold diet by contacting their organization (see Appendix A) or reading Dr. Benjamin Feingold's book, *Why Your Child is Hyperactive*, Random House, 1975. Eliminate salicylates as discussed in Dr. Feingold's material.
- Eliminate refined sugar, food additives, artificial colors, flavors, preservatives, and artificial sweeteners.
- Helpful supplements: liquid calcium and magnesium, choline, vitamin B complex, flaxseed oil, amino acids.
- Help build coordination with planned exercise.
- Chamomile tea at bedtime can be soothing.
- See supplement recommendations (Appendix B).

Constipation and Diarrhea

The frequency and consistency of bowel movements can lead to constipation or diarrhea. "Regular" actually implies having a

[12] Ibid, 173.

bowel movement after each regular meal, not just daily. However, nursed infants do have fewer bowels movements than babies on formula.

Constipation is often caused by too little water, too little fiber, and food allergies. Emotional stress can also cause children to avoid eliminating and thereby create hard stools and constipation. With the added pain of a hard stool, the child avoids the next bowel movement, which starts a cycle of avoidance.

A dirty colon from constipation can lead to many toxic problems, including cancer. A breakdown of the immune system eventually follows extended problems with constipation. This disorder is often called toxic bowel.

On the other extreme is diarrhea or loose/watery stools. Fever, cramping, stomach pain, nausea, and extra thirst may accompany diarrhea. Diarrhea is one of the body's ways of eliminating toxins and other foreign substances.

Diarrhea may be caused by parasites, food poisoning, lack of digestion, allergies, or a virus. In young children, diarrhea can lead to dehydration, if there is a lack of fluid intake.

GENERAL RECOMMENDATIONS

CONSTIPATION

- ••• Increase amount of water and fiber in diet (i.e., fresh fruit, whole grain breads, prunes, cooked prune juice, veggies). Hot cereals, such as oatmeal, can add fiber.
- ••• Check for allergies. Do not introduce solid foods too early. Avoid dairy, wheat, peanuts, yeast, and eggs.
- ••• Include more raw foods and be sure not to overeat.
- ••• Have child get plenty of exercise.
- ••• Determine a better way for child to handle emotional stress. Provide more nurturing.
- ••• Try the introduction of green powders, such as Kyo-Green, mixed with water or added to fruit smoothies.

DIARRHEA

- ••• Fasting, under supervision, can help heal. Often a child will not be hungry and should not be forced to eat.
- ••• Avoid all cold foods.
- ••• Add more fluids to diet.
- ••• Check for food allergies and eliminate dairy.
- ••• Avoid foods that are hard to digest, such as meats. Digestive enzymes may be helpful.
- ••• Eliminate refined sugars and food containing sugar.
- ••• If the diarrhea is antibiotic related, try yogurt without sugar and with live acidophilus cultures.

Obesity

"Obesity is now the leading nutrition problem of all children," according to William Dietz, Ph. D., director of clinical nutrition at the New England Medical Center in Boston. Depending on your source, childhood obesity is estimated at 30% to 50% of school age children.

Weight problems can begin as early as in infants. Many infants are given 70% to 250% more calories than they need. A fat baby often leads to a fat child. Research shows that 75% of children who are overweight between the ages of 9 and 12 will be overweight as adults.[13]

Obesity is when a child weighs 10% more than the average child his age, height, and sex. Overweight comes from too much fuel (energy or calories from food) and too little energy output (exercise). The most obvious culprit is junk food — high calories and minimal nutrition.

Many weight problems and eating disorders stem from emotional problems, habit, or even boredom. Looking at the

[13] Zand, Walton, and Rountree, *Smart Medicine for a Healthier Child*, 320.

emotional roots of a problem can help in resolving the problem. Many excellent books are available covering eating disorders. Get educated on the cause and treatment. Two hotlines that are available are:

- ••• Anorexia Helpline 1-800-888-4673
- ••• Bulimia Abuse Helpline 1-800-888-4680

GENERAL RECOMMENDATIONS

- ••• Develop healthy eating habits.
- ••• Watch out for the beginning of eating disorders.
- ••• Do not focus on weight, but on improving overall health.
- ••• A chromium supplement can often help with sugar cravings, increase metabolic rate, and thereby help with weight loss.
- ••• A digestive enzyme supplement can help with digestion and thereby weight loss.
- ••• Increase water intake to help flush toxins.
- ••• Avoid crash diets or temporary diets. Work on developing healthy lifestyle eating patterns for the whole family.
- ••• Avoid addictive foods, such as sugar, additives, preservatives, chocolate, and caffeine.
- ••• Encourage regular mealtimes and healthy snacks.
- ••• Avoid high fat foods and cooking methods.

HOME HEALTH KIT

Building a home health kit provides a great replacement for the old time "medicine cabinet." Having such a kit prepared before you need it will help during times of emergency. Be sure to keep it in a convenient location, yet out of the reach of small children.

Suggested Contents:

- ••• ace bandage
- ••• Band-aids
- ••• bulb syringe
- ••• hot water bottle
- ••• witch hazel
- ••• scissors with rounded tips
- ••• safety pins
- ••• sterile gauze pads
- ••• adhesive tape
- ••• sterilized needle
- ••• thermometer
- ••• tweezers

Treatment Products, such as:

- ••• aloe vera gel, Mannatech™ Emprisone (for soothing)
- ••• calendula cream
- ••• chamomile and peppermint tea (for digestion and relaxation — Celestial Seasoning's teas are excellent)
- ••• echinacea tincture (for use as a natural antibiotic)
- ••• flaxseed oil (for cell membrane health and skin health)
- ••• mullein/garlic oil (for earaches and ear infections)
- ••• epsom salts (for cleansing and soothing baths)
- ••• drawing salve (for splinters, swollen glands, and boils)
- ••• ginger (for motion sickness)
- ••• ginger or ginger/fennel (for digestion)

CHOOSING THE RIGHT HEALTH CARE PRACTITIONER

Knowing who to select to help you with the care of your child can be a difficult responsibility. The following tips can give you ideas of questions to ask or skills to look for.

- ••• Know the type of skills you want (i.e., traditional medicine, nutritionist, homeopathic, naturopathic, or a combination).
- ••• What are the credentials of the provider? What is his/her schooling and professional experience? Seek a list of referrals.
- ••• How much time does the provider spend with a client? How does the provider interact with children?
- ••• What types of services are offered in the office? Is educational information provided?
- ••• What is the cost of the services provided? Will the provider work with tests from other sources? What is the cost of an initial visit? Are insurance services offered?
- ••• Is the provider compassionate? Caring? Does the caregiver explain what he/she is doing and why?
- ••• Is the provider open to alternative methods of healing?

See Appendix A for names and addresses of alternative health care organizations and other resource organizations.

CHAPTER TEN

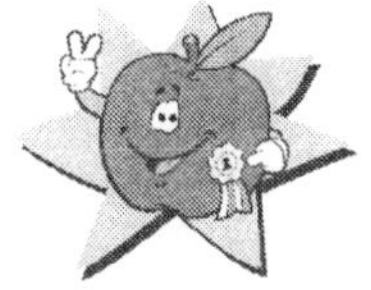

Health is a process that takes time.

You Can Do It!

Are you feeling a little overwhelmed? Do you feel inadequate as a parent? There are times when I see a tremendous gap between what I want to do for our daughter and what I have done. What is that process called? *Guilt*!

It does no good to look at what you haven't done. Feeling guilty only paralyzes a person from moving forward. How can we avoid falling into the guilt trap? Several ways; let's take a look at them.

CHANGE IS A PROCESS

Our family has been progressing in this health process for six years. The key word here is "process." Don't think that health for you or your family will come instantly. Sickness and disease do not happen instantly nor does health. Health is a process that takes time. Give yourself permission to take that time.

It takes time to learn a new way to look at food. It takes time to view physical symptoms as the signs to take better care of the body instead of the sign to take an antibiotic. It takes time to learn to shop differently, prioritize money expenditures differently, cook differently, and eat differently. And, if it takes you time, you know it will also take some time for your children to change.

Health is a process that will last the rest of your life. Today I am amazed at how much I have learned and even more amazed at how much I have yet to learn about health! Our bodies are truly awesomely made. There is much to learn. That is the health process… learning… doing… learning… doing. Anything less is dying.

Since this process will take the rest of your life, enjoy the process and don't just look for the results. If you don't enjoy yourself, you will have missed your life or your child's life. What a sad and expensive price for not learning to enjoy the *process* of getting healthy.

APPLAUD YOUR PROGRESS

It is so easy to see our failures or inadequacies. They often seem to loom larger than life in our eyes. Yet, how much are you already doing that is healthy? Have you made any steps of progress? If you have, then applaud your progress. Encourage yourself to keep moving in that direction.

Have you heard the proverb: You catch more flies with honey than vinegar? That word of wisdom works with you as a parent with yourself as much as with others. Encourage yourself with your progress, instead of beating yourself up over missed opportunities.

If, on the other hand, you really aren't progressing in the area of health, take a minute and determine why. Inventory the situation and identify what can be done in the situation. Then, do it… one step at a time.

ONE STEP AT A TIME

Many times in the early stages of getting healthy, I could only go "5 minutes" more. Those "5 minute" increments were manageable and kept me going. Soon "5 minutes" became 1 hour, 1 day, and 1 year. Today, I have lived through millions of "5 minutes" and I'm much progressed. How exciting! You can do the same in your life.

Today, I encourage you to explore the adventure of getting you and your child (children) healthy. Believe you are on an adventure — you will enjoy your learning curve so much more.

I know you can be a wonderful parent. You have been created to give to your children more than just their birth. You can give them health, which is an inheritance money cannot buy. When you feel a little inadequate, ask our Creator for help. Our Lord is more than willing to be strong when we are weak.

I BLESS YOU WITH…

- ••• wisdom (knowing what to do and when to do it)
- ••• patience (as ingredient every parent needs in abundance!)
- ••• persistence (the willingness to do the right thing day after day after day)

and

- ••• vision (the ability to see your child living out his/her destiny)

Remember, *you* can do it! Just get that extra help from your spiritual Dad. He's got His hand stretched out with the jewels of health. Receive them. *You Can Do It!*

Part Three:

Powerful Alternatives

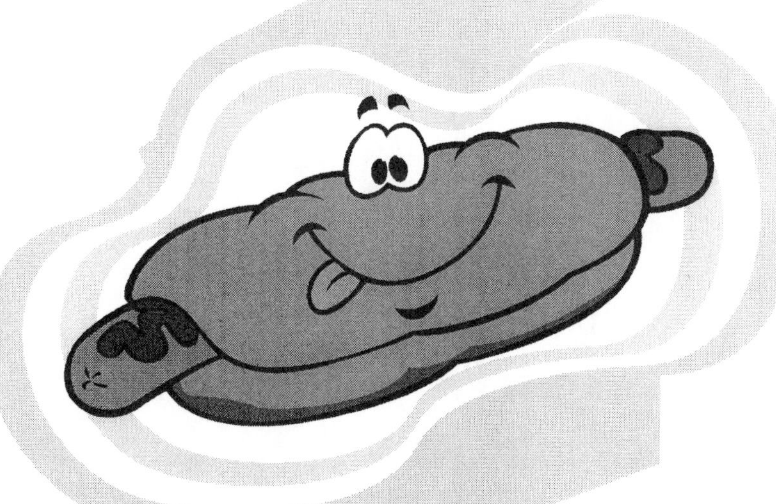

CHAPTER ELEVEN

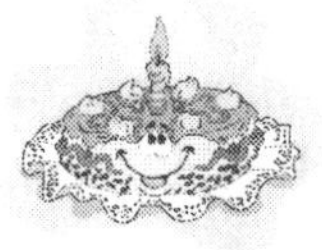

Knowing tasty alternatives to your child's favorite, unhealthy foods makes transition a "piece of cake."

20 Common Foods and Their Healthier Alternatives

What do you do about all of the family favorite foods? Knowing good alternatives, whether you cook or not, can make this dilemma a "piece of cake!" In this chapter, we will walk through the healthier options for:

- cereals
- dairy products
- pancakes, breads, and other breakfast foods
- beverages — including breakfast drinks, sodas, and juices
- packaged lunch items — including soups, pasta meals, applesauce, and pizza
- macaroni and cheese, and hot dogs
- condiments — including ketchup, peanut butter, and jelly
- snacks — including candy, chips, cookies, cakes, and popsicles

As you begin to understand that you do have options as to what you offer to your child, you will begin to grow in confidence. Knowing some healthier options for all of your child's favorite foods is a great relief. If you enjoy cooking, many kid-approved-alternative recipes are given in the *Kid Smart!* recipe section. Or, if you need a quick purchased item to replace the homecooked items, alternative brands are given to help you make an informed choice. Either way, you will be armed with options to unhealthy, fat-laden, sugar-laden, and chemical-laden "foods."

As we walk through these option categories, I will list several brands of each. The first brand will be a nationally recognized brand of traditional "kid-pleasing" food. Listing all of the ingredients in each food will help highlight what is actually contained in this popular brand. My purpose in doing this is not to criticize any one brand, but rather to help you focus on exactly what is in a normal brand of this type of food. These ingredients listed are what most parents are feeding to their children.

Contrast that first ingredient list with the corresponding list found with the healthier brand. Once again, the purpose of this exercise is not merely to highlight a good brand, but also to help you see the various options that are currently available to you in health food stores, some supermarkets, and through mail order.

Let's start our informative journey with a modern morning staple. Yes, I'm speaking of that fabulous favorite of Saturday morning cartoon advertisers everywhere, the ever popular, ever so simple, ever satisfying... breakfast cereal!

CEREALS

Many families routinely start their day with packaged cold cereals. Most regular cereals are heavily laced with sugar, fat, dyes, and various chemicals. In addition, they are also quite expensive — as you may have noticed. Let's take a look at the ingredients of a regular cereal.

Kelloggs Low-Fat Granola
Whole oats, whole wheat, brown sugar, raisins, rice, corn syrup, almonds, glycerin, partially hydrogenated cottonseed or soybean oil, modified corn starch, salt, cinnamon, nonfat dry milk, polyglycerol esters, malt flavoring.

Kellogg's granola contains refined sugar and other non-food items. Do you want your child eating that type of cereal? Let's look at one of the many options.

Breadshop's Granola Strawberry 'n Cream
Rolled oats, grape concentrate, canola oil, freeze-dried strawberries, oat bran, natural strawberry flavor, soy milk powder.

Granola, as with any whole grain cereal, can be a very healthy food. Whole grains are high in the B vitamins, which help us deal with stress. However, once the grains are processed into white flour, we have an ingredient that works in a similar fashion to white sugar.

Homemade granola is actually quite simple to make. Be sure to check out the Crunchy Granola recipe in the Grains Chapter of this book. Changing the dried fruit, seeds, grains, nuts, or sweeteners allow for tremendous variety in the granola. Let your child help you make granola. Encourage him or her to select some of the options and make it "their" cereal. Oftentimes, ownership of the food preparation leads to that food becoming a child's very "favorite." Ownership is always a key to liking something.

Making homemade granola can also become a quick, easy gift for holiday gift giving. Or kids could also have "corner granola sales" (replacing the more well-known lemonade stands). Making, selling, or giving homemade granola is a great homeschool or family activity.

If you want an alternative to your traditional packaged cereal, I recommend the following brands:

Cold Cereals
Health Valley Fat Free Granola
Back To Nature Granola
Breadshop's Granola
Golden Temple Granola
Life Stream Granola

The following list gives you some ideas of alternatives to specific traditional cereals. If you think your child might resist a new brand, have a transition plan. For example, if your child just loves Fruit Loops (loaded with dyes, sugar, white flour, preservatives), mix a small amount of the new cereal with the old. Slowly increase the proportion of the new cereal. Soon, they will be eating only the new. This technique can work with milks and many other foods.

Cheerios	Oatios (both plain and Honey 'n Almond) Nature O's Barbara's Breakfast O's
Kix	Pure & Simple puffed cereals Arrowhead Mills Nature Puffs Erewhon Poppets
Corn Flakes	Arrowhead Mills Kamut Flakes Barbara's Corn Flakes Erewhon Organic Wheat Flakes

	Health Valley Amaranth Flakes Nature's Path Brown Rice Flakes or Corn Flakes
Rice Krispies	Barbara's Brown Rice Crispies Erewhon Crispy Brown Rice Health Valley Crisp Rice
Raisin Bran	Erewhon Organic Raisin Bran Health Valley Raisin Bran Nature's Path Manna Flakes Raisin Nature's Path Millet Rice Flakes
Fruit Loops	Health Valley Bran O's Fruit New Morning Fruit-E-O's New Morning Apple Cinnamon Oatios
Grape Nuts	Perky's Nutty Rice
Muesli	Rhine Harvest Muesli

In addition to these cold cereals, there are many wonderful, nutritious hot cereals on the market. You can now find instant, whole grain cup-a-cereals. These instant cereals are great for travel, baby-sitters, and other times when "quick" is the key word. Some of the whole grain, natural hot cereals now on the market include:

Hot Cereals
Erewhon
The Grain Place
Lundberg Hot n' Creamy
Arrowhead Mills
Montana's Cream of the West
Fantastic Foods
American Prairie
Bob's Red Mill

DAIRY PRODUCTS

We have already discussed the many potential problems of milk and other dairy products. There are so many commercial and homemade options to dairy products today that you will never miss dairy — or the resulting mucus.

Our *Lifestyle for Health* cookbook has an entire section of milk and all of the possible dairy products and their many options. Please refer to it for a full array of substitution options. Here, we will look at the basic area of milk as both a beverage and a cooking ingredient.

Many options are now available for cow's milk. Some children do better with goat's milk. Finding raw goat's milk from a clean, local source can be difficult. If you can it is often an option for babies, as well as children. The canned goat's milk that I have tried is not very tasty, and most children dislike it.

Some of the easiest alternatives to dairy milk are rice, soy, and almond. Most of the commercial milk alternatives come in boxes or aseptic packaging. These boxes have pour spouts and are quite convenient to store in your pantry until opened. Once opened, they should be stored in the refrigerator and used within five days.

Most brands are available in both 8 ounce (individual servings) and quart sizes. They come in many flavors, depending on their intended use. The 8 ounce size is great for travel (use with one of the instant, whole grain cereals for a nutritious, yet quick, hot meal in hotels or while on the road traveling).

Rice milk is usually made from the starch portion of brown rice. It is considered less allergenic than soy. It is wise to rotate your milks, if your family tends toward allergies. Rice milk can be made at home. See the beverage chapter for a recipe. Rice milk works well in sauces and in baking (i.e., muffins, breads, cakes, etc).

Soy milk is made from soybeans. It is usually a little richer, even the lite versions, than rice milk. Soy milk makes a richer sauce, gravy, or pudding than rice milk. It bakes better in baked puddings than rice milk, which can separate. See the beverage chapter for a recipe for homemade soy milk.

For children who are allergic to grains, almond milk can be a wonderful option. Almonds are naturally high in calcium, low in fat, and one of the easiest nuts to digest. Almond milk is easy to make, or it can be purchased. Wholesome and Hearty has ready-made almond milk. They also have some excellent cheeses and frozen entrees.

You can also make milk or "cream" from cashews and oats. I know of no commercial brands of cashew or oat milks. However, recipes can be found in the beverage chapter.

When looking for alternative cheeses, Rella is a brand that I prefer. It melts well and it comes in varieties from cheddar to Monterrey Jack and mozzarella, to name only a few.

Some of our favorite alternative milk brands include:

Rice Milk
Rice Dream by Imagine Foods
Westbrae Natural Foods
Pacific Foods of Oregon
Health Valley

Soy Milk
Eden Foods
Westbrae Natural Food
VitaSoy

Almond Milk
Wholesome and Hearty

Tofu
Sovex Better Than Milk?

Amazake*
Grainaissance

* Amazake is both a brand and a form of rice milk. It is made from the whole brown rice grain. Other rice milks use only the starch portion, which allows for a more white-colored beverage. Amazake is thicker and darker in color. It is more nutritious. It

can be diluted with half water (pure) for a young child's beverage or for cooking. Amazake can also be used as an egg replacer (approximately 1/4 cup of amazake for 1 egg).

PANCAKES, BREADS AND OTHER BREAKFAST FOODS

Common alternatives to cereal for the average American includes pancakes, waffles, toast, and pop tarts. Once again, many of these foods are loaded with sugar, fat, white flour, dyes, and preservatives. This is not a very nutritious way to start you or your child's day.

Let's take a look at some of the traditional brands and their ingredients.

Aunt Jemima Pancake Mix
Enriched flour, sugar, rice flour, sodium bicarbonate, sodium aluminum phosphate, salt.

Compare Aunt Jemima's ingredients to those found in a mix by Arrowhead Mills.

Arrowhead Mills Oat Bran Pancake Mix
Organic oat bran, organic whole wheat flour, organic wheat bran, buttermilk solids, non-aluminum baking powder, potassium bicarbonate.

The sodium content in Aunt Jemima is 620 mg. and Arrowhead Mills is 260 mg. That difference is significant and one to consider if pancakes are part of your regular diet. Other brands of pancake mix include David's Goodbatter and Bob's Red Mill, Pamela's, VitaSpelt by Purity Foods, Maple Grove Farms of Vermont.

The grains chapter gives you several recipes for pancakes and waffles. Our family often makes extra pancakes and/or waffles on weekends. We freeze the extras. During the week, Anna pops the extras (which were undercooked) in the toaster. In moments she has a hot, wholesome, inexpensive pancake or waffle. This makes week-day breakfasts a snap.

Most of the syrups used to cover pancakes and waffles contain refined sugar, dyes, and preservatives. Pure maple syrup is a healthier option to these other syrups. In the snack chapter you will find recipes for other alternatives to these sugar-laden syrups. They are quite delicious, easy to make, and inexpensive options.

If you want a frozen waffle, once again you have alternatives. A well known frozen brand of waffles has the following ingredients:

Kellogg's Eggo Waffles
Enriched wheat flour, egg whites, sugar, water, baking soda, sodium aluminum phosphate, monocalcium phosphate, potassium chloride, salt, artificial flavors, spice, beta carotene.

In comparison, Van's uses the following ingredients:

Van's 7 Grain Frozen Belgian Waffles
Water, whole wheat flour, canola oil, pear, pineapple, peach sweetener, yeast, lecithin, natural vanilla, rye flour, barley flour, rice flour, yellow corn flour, soy flour, sea salt.

Van's also has gluten-free and wheat-free frozen waffles. They are actually quite tasty.

In addition to pancakes and waffles, some children eat Pop Tarts. Let's take a look at the ingredient list of this breakfast delight.

Kellogg's Cherry Pop Tart
Filling: Corn syrup, dextrose, high fructose corn syrup, crackermeal, modified corn starch, dried cherries, citric acid, xanthan gum, red #10 natural flavor, blue #1 natural flavor.

Crust: Enriched wheat flour, sugar, soybean oil, high fructose corn syrup, salt, leavening, sodium stearoyl lactylate, diacetyl tartaric acid, esters of mono and diglycerides.

Few of these ingredients provide any nutrition. The one or two healthier options that I have found in health food stores have never had any flavor. Instead of a pop tart, how about a piece of toast with jam? The nutrition content is much higher while the fat and chemical content is much lower.

However, when looking at bread, not all breads are the same. White bread obviously contains white flour. Are you aware of what else it contains? Look at the following contents of the popular Iron Kids Bread:

Rainbo Iron Kids Bread

Enriched flour, water, high fructose corn syrup, soy hull fiber, wheat gluten, yeast, partially hydrogenated soybean oil, salt, soy flour, dough conditioners, yeast nutrients, amylase, cornstarch, calcium propionate.

If you want another example of just how void of nutrition white bread is, try the following experiment. Take a loaf of whole grain bread and a loaf of white bread. Placing a hand on each end of the loaf, push toward the center. Do this to both loaves in turn. You will see that the white loaf will squish to a small doughy mush. The whole grain loaf (if totally made from whole grain flours) will indent only slightly and return to its original shape.

A whole grain bread would have the following type of ingredient list:

Rudi's Honey Whole Wheat Bread

Stone ground whole wheat flour, purified water, raw honey, organic canola oil, vital wheat gluten, salt, yeast, lecithin, may contain some vinegar.

Most whole grain breads are unique to a region. In the Rocky Mountain Region, I recommend Great Harvest Bread. Their products are made from freshly milled flours, which have the natural oils still fresh. This is whole grain in its richest, most nutritional form and the most tasty.

National brands, such as French Meadow and Pacific Bakery, provide whole-grain breads, as well as yeast-free and wheat-free options. In addition to bread, be sure to check out options such as tortillas and pita breads. These healthier brands include the following:

Whole Wheat Tortillas
Laariposa
Garden of Eatin'
Stacey's
Leopoldo's

White Flour Tortillas
Brooke Rose Vegetable Tortillas
Stacey's
Leona's

Pita Bread
Garden of Eatin'
Rudi's
Food for Life

BEVERAGES

PROTEIN DRINKS

Beverages go beyond breakfast and on into the rest of the day. However, before we leave breakfast foods, let's look at protein drinks. Many people, especially teens and athletes, drink protein power drinks for breakfast. Let's look at a well-known protein drink and its ingredients.

Carnation Vanilla Instant Breakfast
Nonfat dry milk, maltodextrin, sugar, cellulose, gum, natural vanilla flavor.

Are there alternatives that are as quick and easy? Yes! Many protein drinks can be found in health food stores. When selecting one, be sure to check the ingredient list. Shaklee has a protein drink that is quite tasty, without the refined sugar and preservatives. Other alternatives are Nature's Plus, Nature's Life, Solgar, and The Ultimate Life.

Naturade Vanilla N-R-G Protein Drink

Isolated soy protein, calcium caseinate, whey protein concentrate, enzymatically predigested lactalbumin, egg albumen, lecithin, papain (papaya enzyme), carrageenan (sea kelp), natural flavors.

A great alternative to these protein drinks (which are often fairly expensive) is a fruit smoothie. This has become our breakfast beverage of choice. It is easy and we can load it with nutrition. Best of all, Anna never knows just how nutritious it is (unless she watches us make it). A fruit smoothie has a little more substance (as much as we want it to have) than fruit and thereby makes a more filling breakfast. Many recipes are available in the beverage chapter.

When making your own fruit smoothie, consider adding some of the following supplements for added nutritional punch:

KyoGreen — this is our favorite green powder. Green superfoods provide vitamins, minerals, protein, and enzymes in an easily absorbed form. They also tend to gently cleanse and neutralize excess acid in the system.

Lecithin (we use Lewis Laboratory brand) — which is good for brain functioning, lubrication of the body, and also for weight distribution.

Brewers' yeast (we use Lewis Laboratory brand) — which is rich in chromium (sugar metabolism, reduction of sugar craving, and increased energy levels).

Flaxseed oil (we recommend Spectrum or Rohé) — which provides essential fatty acids for cell membrane and skin health.

Garlic (we recommend Kyolic) — which is good for immune support and circulatory health.

Acidophilus (we recommend Kyolic or Metagenics) — which is good when you have been on antibiotics or to help bring the intestinal flora/bacteria back into balance.

There are numerous other possibilities of additions. The above are our staple additions to the fruit smoothie recipes found in the beverage chapter. Check the supplementation chapter for additional information on supplements, brands, and dosages by age group.

SODAS

One of the most common beverages consumed by children is soda. Have you recently looked at a can of Classic Coke?

One can contains:

Classic Coke

Carbonated water, high fructose corn syrup and/or sucrose, caramel color, phosphoric acid, natural flavors, caffeine.

Maybe you think you are doing better, avoiding caffeine, and drinking sodas such as 7-Up. Let's look at its ingredients:

7-Up

Carbonated water, high fructose corn syrup and/or sugar, citric acid, sodium citrate, and natural lemon and lime flavors.

Most sugar sweetened sodas contain, on the average, seven teaspoons of sugar per can. This is a tremendous amount of sugar, let alone the caffeine, artificial coloring, and artificial flavorings. However, as much as I dislike sugar, the artificial sweeteners are a less desirable alternative.

Healthier sodas are readily available. Let's look at one such soda brand.

R. W. Knudsen's Spritzer
(Mango Fadango Flavor)
Sparkling water, concentrated white grape juice, mango puree, concentrated passion fruit juice, natural flavors.

Knudsen's spritzers are fruit based with no dyes or sugar. They are healthier, but obviously still not quite as good as old fashioned pure water. Knudsen's, along with other brands, such as After the Fall, BlueSky, Corr's, Dr Tima, Ginseng Up, Hansen, Health Valley, Natural Brew, Reed's Originals, Santa Cruz Naturals, and Tianfu have many flavors of natural sodas. Be sure to read the labels, since even some of these use corn syrup, which is a refined sugar.

FRUIT JUICES
In addition to sodas, a commonly consumed beverage is fruit juice (often *fruit* in name only). Many fruit juices contain little, if any, real fruit juice and are usually high in refined sugar, dyes, and preservatives. Since many children take the small aseptically packaged boxes of juice, let's compare two of these juices. First, lets look at an ever-so-familiar Hi C drink.

Orange Hi C Drink
Water, high fructose corn syrup, sugar, orange juice from concentrate, malic and citric acid, potassium citrate, natural flavorings, ascorbic acid, yellow #6.

Compare this to a box of Knudsen's healthier juice:

R. W. Knudsen's Apple Cranberry Juice
Pressed apple juice, concentrated cranberry juice, natural flavors.

Knudsen's is not the only brand available in this popular food niche. Other healthy, yet delicious, kid approved brands include After the Fall, AME, Mountain Sun, Muir Glen (vegetable juice), and Santa Cruz. In the frozen department, healthier brands include Cascadian Farms, Ferraro's (vegetable and fruit), and Knudsen's.

KOOL AID

One of the only foods for which there is no direct alternative is Kool Aid. My advice to you is that if you are offering Kool Aid to your children for convenience and thrift, consider plain old pure water.

Kool Aid contains the following ingredients:

Kool Aid

Citric acid, calcium phosphate, maltodextrin, salt, natural flavor, lemon juice, ascorbic acid, titanium dioxidy, yellow 5 lake, yellow 5, BHA.

Does your child really need a daily dose of those ingredients? Fruit juices (commercial or fresh) or pure water are far superior. My recommendation for Kool Aid is to stop buying it.

HOT CHOCOLATE

Last, but not least, we can't overlook hot chocolate. What is a cold winter evening without a mug of steaming hot chocolate? Many hot chocolate mixes cantain high levels of caffeine and sugar that can really hype most children. Look at the following ingredients in a familiar hot chocolate mix:

Hershey's Hot Chocolate Milk Mix

Sugar, cocoa, caramel color, cornstarch, salt, carrageenan, soya lecithin, vanillin, dextrin, artificial color red #40, yellow #5, blue #1, sulfur dioxide.

Compare the Hershey's Hot Chocolate Mix ingredient list to that of a healthier brand.

Newmarket Foods Instant Chocolate Milk Mix
Dehydrated molasses and honey, unsweetened dutch process cocoa, soy lecithin, pure vanilla, natural flavors.

The lack of dyes and chemicals is noticeable. Homemade chocolate or carob syrup for instant hot chocolate is very simple to make. Check out the recipe in the beverage chapter. Carob can be used in place of chocolate to eliminate the caffeine. Soy, rice, or almond milks can be used to eliminate all of the dairy. What a treat. It is so easy, a child could make it.

In addition to all of those options, many of the packaged soy, almond, and rice milks are available in chocolate and carob flavors. These milks can be heated for another instant version of hot chocolate.

PACKAGED LUNCH ITEMS

As we pass the breakfast time of day, we move into lunch or dinner. Many parents buy convenient boxed or frozen foods, oblivious to their contents. When I did the research for this book and investigated the ingredients of these foods, I was aghast. What a tray of poisons to feed to a small (or big) child's body. It's time to wake up to the multitude of options that are easy, tasty, and far healthier.

SOUPS

Chicken and noodle soup is a common lunch for many children, especially when they are sick. Campbell's has been a mother's helper for generations. However, our daughter, having not grown up eating canned soups, finds most of them fairly tasteless, as do her parents. There are some acceptable convenience soups; Campbell's is not one I would recommend. Why?

For starters, let's take a look at exactly what's in Campbell's Chicken Noodle Soup.

Campbell's Chicken Noodle Soup
Chicken stock, enriched egg noodles, chicken, carrots, water, salt, margarine, potato starch, celery, MSG, chicken fat, yeast extract, onion powder, vegetable oil, dehydrated parsley, modified food starch, sodium phosphates, soy protein, chicken flavor, dehydrated garlic, flavoring, citric acid.

We would not want a food with margarine, MSG, yeast, and commercial chicken.

Compare this to a can of Shelton's chicken noodle soup. Shelton's uses natural chickens that are raised without any hormones and chemicals.

Shelton's Chicken Noodle Soup
Water, chicken, carrots, whole wheat egg noodles, onions, chicken broth, celery, potato starch, sea salt, chicken fat, dried garlic, spices, parsley.

Many packaged healthier soups exist, from instant to canned to bean mixes for crockpot use. Some of our favorite brands include Muir (tomato), Hain, Bearito, Health Valley, Fantastic Foods, Westbrae, and The Spice Hunter.

PASTA MEALS

Do your children like the old, familiar Chef Boyardee meals? Have you checked out the ingredients? Let's look at them.

Chef Boyardee Spaghetti and Meat Balls
Tomatoes, water, cooked enriched spaghetti, beef, high fructose corn syrup, crackermeal, salt, modified food starch, enriched wheat flour, soy protein isolate, onions, MSG, hydrolyzed corn, soy, wheat protein, caramel coloring, flavorings, modified cheese.

I have not found a tasty, canned alternative to this interesting mixture. However, several frozen entrees might fill the bill. Brands worth checking out include Amy's, Cascadian Farm, and Ken & Robert's. Several recipes for pasta meals can also be found in the main dish chapter.

APPLESAUCE

Very few kids dislike applesauce. However, even such a simple food can have added, unnecessary ingredients if you select certain manufacturers. Let's look at what one company has done to this simple food.

Musselman's

Apples, corn syrup, sugar, water, erythorbic acid.

Compared to the healthier alternatives, Musselman's has more added sugar than is necessary.

Santa Cruz

Apples.

Other brands of healthier applesauce include Solana Gold, Cherry Hill, and Skyland. Several of these brands also have a variety of flavor combinations. Check out their many terrific combinations and add a little variety to your child's applesauce. Most of these brands are available in individual servings as well as larger containers.

PIZZA

Pizza has become an American favorite. The primary choice seems to be pepperoni pizza with lots of extra cheese. We already know the danger of those two ingredients. But wait, that's not all you get with these all-American taste treats, there's more! Let's take a look at the other questionable ingredients added to the average frozen pizza.

Tombstone Pepperoni Pizza
Topping: Part skim mozzarella, brick cheese, tomato paste, pepperoni (pork, beef, salt, water, dextrose, spices, lactic acid starter, oleoresin of paprika, flavoring).

Compare this to a healthier, frozen pizza, such as Graindance Whole Wheat pizza.

Graindance Whole Wheat Cheese Pizza
Organic whole wheat flour, water, yeast, unrefined safflower and corn oil, unfiltered honey, sea salt, molasses, tomato puree, tomatoes, soybean oil, onion, salt, olive oil, romano cheese, fresh herbs, pure spices.

Other healthier brands include Original Rice Crust Pizza, Ken & Robert's (pocket pizza), and Wolfgang Puck. A great recipe is included in the main dish chapter of this book for both vegetarian pizza and pizza crust. Try them, experimenting with almost any topping you can imagine. They freeze well and are easy to make. Pizzas have always been one of the biggest hits in my cooking classes.

Pizza parties are a great way to entertain kids at birthday parties — young or old. Make the crust in individual serving sizes ahead of time (they can be frozen). Have lots of topping options (healthy, of course). Then, when the time comes, have the children make their own pizzas. Often, they will even try some of the vegetable toppings. This has been a hit at our house for years!

Another easy option for a quick pizza is to use split pita bread or a tortilla for the crust. Cover it with sauce and your own choice of healthy and delicious toppings. The Rella brand of soy and almond cheese melts well and is a great dairy-free addition to these quick pizzas. If your child resists, just mix a dairy cheese half and half with the soy. Soon, they will never notice the difference.

MACARONI AND CHEESE

Another childhood favorite is macaroni and cheese or "cheese and macaroni." The most popular brand of this food seems to be Kraft, so let's take a look at their ingredient choices.

Kraft Macaroni and Cheese

Enriched macaroni, cheese sauce, water, whey protein concentrate, skim milk, salt, buttermilk, sodium phosphate, citric acid, yellow #5, yellow #6, lactic acid.

In addition to these ingredients, one serving (3/4 cup) of Kraft macaroni and cheese contains a very high level of sodium. An alternative pasta product, DeBoles Shells and Cheddar, contains much less sodium and healthier ingredients without sacrificing taste.

DeBoles Pasta and Cheese

Durum semolina and artichoke flour, cheddar cheese, whey, sweetcream buttermilk.

VitaSpelt has also introduced a macaroni and cheese product using spelt flour. Many people that are sensitive to wheat can use spelt flour products. This may be an alternative for you.

Of course, you could always do it yourself. To make macaroni and cheese yourself, simply cook a pasta that works for your family (i.e., corn, spelt, kamut, etc.). Melt a soy (almond or raw milk) cheese with a small amount of rice (or whole wheat) flour. Stir in milk (soy, almond, or rice), along with the cooked pasta. Season with garlic salt or tamari. It is easy, inexpensive, and quite tasty.

HOT DOGS

The American pastime of an afternoon (or evening) at a ball game traditionally includes... hot dogs! Though ever popular, hot dogs can be a terribly chemically-laden "food." Let's look at one of the most popular hot dog brands and see what ingredients they contain.

Ball Park Hot Dog

Beef and pork, turkey, water, dextrose, salt, corn syrup, flavorings, hydrolyzed beef stock, sodium phosphates, sodium nitrite, extractives of paprika, ascorbic acid.

The nitrites are quite toxic to children. If you choose to feed your child this "food," at least follow it with a megadose of vitamin C to help boost the immune system to deal with it. A better "hot dog" choice would be to select a healthier turkey dog (one made from natural turkey) or one of the available vegetarian options.

Some of the many tasty, vegetarian dogs include Lightlife, White Wave, and Soy Boy Not Dogs. Let's look at what all they contain.

Soy Boy Not Dogs

Organic tofu, isolated soy protein, tapioca flour, yeast extracts, corn oil, yeast, onion powder, garlic powder, herbs, spices, dried molasses, vegetable flavorings, vegetable gum, sea salt.

Lightlife Wonderdogs

Water, isolated soy protein, vital wheat gluten, natural flavors from vegetable sources, soy oil, sea salt, rice syrup solids, spice extracts, paprika, oleoresin, carageenan, vegetable gums.

Shelton's Turkey Franks

Turkey, water, sea salt, mustard, spices.

Vegetarian patties are also hitting the market. One of our all-time favorites is Boca Burgers. Add this patty to a whole grain bun, with toppings of lettuce, tomato, and ketchup and you have a real taste treat.

CONDIMENTS (KETCHUP, PEANUT BUTTER, AND JELLY)

KETCHUP

When you add an inconspicuous condiment like ketchup, most people never think twice about its impact on health. Yet, many ketchups have a high level of sugar. Hunt's is a familiar brand, let's look at their ingredient list.

Hunt's Ketchup

Tomato concentrate, high fructose corn syrup, distilled vinegar, corn syrup, salt, onion powder, garlic powder, natural flavors.

Compare this toWestbrae's ingredient list.

Westbrae Natural Catsup

Tomato paste, water, white grape juice, cider vinegar, onion powder, natural flavor.

Muir has come out with a ketchup in a plastic container more like traditional ketchups. The taste is superb, which makes it another great alternative. When you add that ketchup to a hot dog or patty, be sure you are putting all of it into a whole grain bun. The whole grain bun adds many B vitamins and fiber not found in white bread.

PEANUT BUTTER

A busy mom's standby is a PBJ sandwich. Although this is not one of my favorite sandwiches, most kids seem to inhale these sandwiches. Let's take a look at what some companies add to the basic ingredient of peanuts.

Peter Pan Peanut Butter

Roasted peanuts, sugar, partially hydrogenated vegetable oil, salt.

Compare this to a healthier alternative.

Roaster Fresh Peanut Butter
Peanuts.

Peanut butter should be this simple. In fact, if you have a good quality blender (i.e., Bosch), you can make your own peanut butter or other nut butters. They are quite tasty and fresh. Other health-oriented brands of nut butters include Maranatha, Toner, Arrowhead Mills, Spanky's, and Adams.

Other nut butters can be used in place of peanut butter. Almond butter is lower in fat, easier to digest, and higher in calcium than peanut butter. Other options include cashew hazelnut, sesame (or tahini), and sunflower butter.

Once again, vary your foods to prevent allergies. Our daughter ate a steady diet of PBJ sandwiches for a period of time and developed a peanut allergy. Rotating your nuts can help prevent such an allergy from occurring.

JELLY

Most jellies are nothing but sugar, water, and maybe juice. Let's check out some ingredients.

Welch's Grape Jelly
Grapes, corn syrup, high fructose corn syrup, fruit pectin, citric acid, sodium citrate.

Instead of sugar-rich jellies, try some of the new fruit-only jams. They are tastier and contain less refined sugar.

Cascadian Farm Organic Spreadable Fruit
Organic grape juice concentrate, organic concord grapes, fruit pectin, citric acid.

Cascadian is an excellent choice, due to its commitment to organic ingredients. Other brands of jam are R. W. Knudsen, American Spoon, McCutcheon's, Sorrell Ridge, Wagner's, and Kozlowski Farms.

SNACKS

CANDY

One of the most popular candies today seems to be M&M's. These artificially colored, sugar-laden morsels are anything but healthy. Let's look at the ingredients of M&M's.

M&M's

Milk chocolate (first ingredient of milk chocolate is sugar), sugar, cornstarch, corn syrup, gum acacia, red #40, yellow #6, yellow #5, blue #1, dextrin.

Can you believe there is actually a healthier alternative to M&M's? Sunspire is a company that makes chocolate candies (and chocolate chips, as well as carob candies) without refined sugar, preservatives, and food dyes. Sunspire also has seasonal candies (Valentine, Easter, Christmas, etc.) in both chocolate and carob.

Sunspire Sun Drops

Dried cane juice and unsulphured molasses, whole milk powder, cocoa butter, unsweetened chocolate, soy lecithin, vanilla, turbinado sugar, whole rice solids, beet juice, beta carotene, caramel, vegetable and bee's wax, food glaze (no sugar).

Another excellent company that provides tasty, sugar-free candy is FruitSource. They have delicious chocolate covered tidbits such as nuts, maltballs, and pretzels.

If you prefer candy bars, try Tropical Source. They have large and bite sized chocolates, made without refined sugar, preservatives, and dyes.

Queen Bee is a line of gourmet candies, including truffles. They have a carob line and all are made with honey instead of refined sugar. They make great gift items.

In addition to chocolate, licorice and gummy bears are favorite candies. Let's look at what is contained in gummy bears.

Gummy Bears

Corn syrup, sugar gelatin, citric acid, natural and artificial flavor, artificial color, FD&C blue #1, yellow #5, #6, red #40, vegetable oil, carnauba wax.

Instead of gummy bears, let's look at an alternative licorice-type candy.

Panda Licorice Chews

Molasses, wheat flour, licorice extract, anise seed oil.

If you choose to give your child candy, at least make it as healthy a candy as possible. Lots of sugar, dyes, and artificial ingredients on a regular basis, or even just during the holidays, is not helping your child. There are so many tasty options that you can easily help your child in this area, without sacrificing taste buds.

COOKIES

Even when candy is not considered, cookies often are. As we have changed our diet and introduced whole grains and natural sweeteners, we have found that one cookie will satisfy our sweet tooth. In the past, a sugar-intense cookie set off cravings for at least a dozen more. The sugar in the first cookie never satisfied and I would find myself, or our daughter, eating a whole package. Believe it or not, the more natural cookies do not have that addictive effect on us. Let's look at a favorite sugar cookie.

Teddy Grahams

Enriched wheat flour, riboflavin, sugar, vegetable shortening, honey, graham flour, baking soda, salt, maltodextrin, soy lecithin.

Yes, there are even alternatives to these cookies. Let's look at the healthier ingredients.

Westbrae Dino Snaps

Organic whole wheat flour, fruit juice concentrate, butter, soy lecithin, natural vanilla, expelled pressed canola oil, baking soda, sea salt, baking powder, natural flavors.

Another of our favorite brands is Pamela's. They are wheat-free, sugar-free, and never use artificial ingredients. They have cookies and brownie mixes. All of their products are truly delicious. Other excellent brands include Barbara's, Westbrae, Carissa's, Frookies, Health Valley, Jennie's, and Mrs. Densons.

CAKES

When birthdays roll around, many people purchase a cake or make a mix. There are alternative recipes and mixes that can produce a delicious cake even the pickiest of children will enjoy. Several recipes can be found for cake and frosting in the dessert chapter of this book and our other cookbooks (*Lifestyle for Health* cookbook and *Meals in 30 Minutes*). Let's look at the familiar Pillsbury cake mix.

Pillsbury White Cake Mix

Sugar, bleached flour, hydrogenated vegetable oil, baking soda, soda aluminum phosphate, wheat starch, modified corn starch, dextrose, propylene glycol, mono and diestres of fatty acids, nono and diglycerides, salt, whey protein concentrate, artificial color, xanthan gum, cellulose gum, guar gum, citric acid polysorbate 60, soy lecithin.

Not many cake mixes (there are more brownie and cookie mixes) are available in health food stores, but I did find one. *Which one do you want?*

Martha's Chocolate Cake Mix

Unbleached flour, sugar, imported Dutch cocoa, aluminum free baking powder, baking soda.

Although it contains sugar, the remaining ingredients are reasonably pure.

Fearn Banana Cake Mix

Stoneground whole wheat pastry flour, soya powder, yogurt solids, dehydrated banana, whey powder, baking soda, salt, cinnamon, natural banana flavor.

ICE CREAM

What is cake, or any dessert, without ice cream? Once again, many alternatives exist. From sugar-free to dairy-free, options abound. Let's take a look at the popsicle versions of ice cream, which seems to be a favorite with most kids.

Snickers Ice Cream Bar

Ice cream: skim milk, cream, sugar corn syrup, peanut butter, cocoa powder, gelatin, mono and diglycerides, carob bean gum, guar gum, salt, carrageenan.
Coating: sugar, cocoa butter, milk, chocolate, lactose, milkfat, soy lecithin, vanillin, coconut oil.
Caramel: corn syrup, milk, sugar, butter, salt, carrageenan, vanillin, peanuts.

One of our favorite variations that has no refined sugar or dairy is Rice Dream. Let's look at their ingredients.

Rice Dream Nutty Bar

Chocolate rice dream: water, partially milled brown rice, expeller safflower oil, cocoa, carob bean, guar gum, carrageenan, soy lecithin, sea salt.
Coating: peanuts, barley and corn malt, coconut oil, unsweetened chocolate, cocoa butter, lecithin, vanilla.

A simple way to have healthy popsicles at home is to make them yourselves. Extra fruit smoothies can easily be frozen in popsicle containers or small paper cups (use craft sticks for handles). Simply peel the paper away and eat the paper-filled popsicles as a quick, easy treat.

Are there alternatives to normal, child-loved food? Yes, there are many. Some you will enjoy more than others, but I believe you will be pleasantly surprised with virtually all of these alternatives. The key is to start making changes somewhere. We have listed brands that our family likes, to help make your adventure into health food as enjoyable as possible. Take advantage of the wonderful products on the market and the delicious recipes in this book and others to help build a healthy child in your family.

Better Beverages

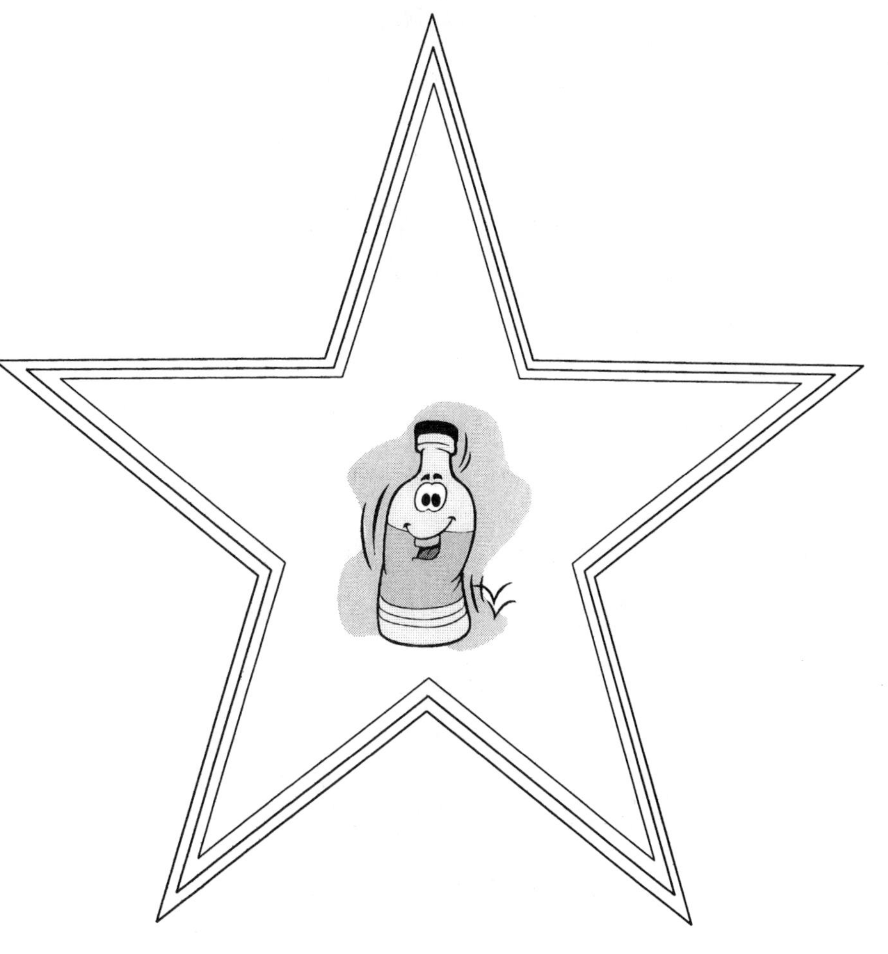

Fruit Smoothie
Fruit Shakes
Almond Milk
Strawberry Milk
Banana Milk
Apple Milk
Strawberry Shake
Peach Shake
Banana Shake
Carob Chip Shake
Carob or Chocolate Syrup
Hot Chocolate
Oat Milk
Rice (or Soy) Milk
Cashew Cream

Fruit Smoothie

This beverage is our daily stand-by. It is more filling than plain fruit juice. Try the many options and then create some of your own. To make all of the options requires a blender and a juicer. A juicer becomes necessary to provide fresh, tasty juices. However, if you are not at that point, use a quality brand of processed juice.

Basic Smoothie Recipe

2 frozen bananas, peeled, cut into chunks (peel frozen bananas by placing under hot water, until the peel removes easily)
1 cup fresh berries, such as strawberries or raspberries
2 cups apple juice

DIRECTIONS:

Blend in blender.

NOTES:

Variations:

- ☆ 2 frozen bananas, 1 cup strawberries, 2 cups pineapple juice
- ☆ 2 frozen bananas, 1 cup strawberries, 2 cups pineapple juice, 2 Tbl. sunflower seeds, 2 Tbl. sesame seeds
- ☆ 2 fresh bananas, 1 cup strawberries, 2 cups orange juice
- ☆ 2 cups apple juice, 1 large sweet apple, 2 pitted dates, 2 frozen bananas, 2 Tbl. sunflower seeds
- ☆ 2 cups apple or orange juice, 2 frozen bananas, 2 ripe peaches (seeded, cut into chunks)

These variations are only a beginning. Add sunflower or sesame seeds (they have 10 times the calcium of milk), lecithin granules (considered an arthritis inhibitor), flaxseed oil (key source of essential fatty acids), and/or pysillium husks (key to regular bowel movement). Many of these additions (in small amounts) do not affect the taste of the beverage and are a good way to add healthful nutrients to your body.

Serves 2 – 3.

Calories: 244 • Protein: (g) 2 • Carbs: (g) 61 • Fat: (g) 1 • Sat. Fat: (g) 0 • Cholesterol: (mg) 0 • Fiber: (g) 5 • Sodium: (mg) 9

Fruit Shakes

A simple, yet tasty drink. Experiment with all kinds of fruits.

- 1 pkg. Mori Nu Tofu, soft
- 2 bananas, frozen
- 3/4 cup rice milk
- 1 cup strawberries, frozen

DIRECTIONS:

Blend all ingredients in blender until smooth.

Serves 2 – 3.

Calories: 225 • Protein: (g) 16 • Carbs: (g) 28 • Fat: (g) 7 •
Sat. Fat: (g) 0 • Cholesterol: (mg) 0 • Fiber: (g) 6 • Sodium: (mg) 16

Almond Milk

Almond Milk is great by itself and as a dairy substitute. It is easy to make in the blender. Since it is not homogenized it, will break down if boiled intensely. It is great over cereal or over fruit salads.

1/2 cup shelled raw almonds*
2 cups water

DIRECTIONS:

1. Place almonds in blender and grind to a fine powder.
2. Add 1 cup water and blend. Add additional cup of water and blend to form a smooth milk.
3. A couple of teaspoons of maple syrup or rice syrup may be added for a sweeter beverage.

NOTES:

* Blanched almonds produce a whiter and smoother beverage. Almonds can be blanched by placing them in 1 cup boiling water. Allow them to stand in the water until the skin easily slips off. Remove skins.

☆ Almonds are an excellent source of protein, B vitamins, essential minerals, unsaturated fats, and fiber. They also contain calcium.

☆ There is a prepackaged Almond Milk available in health food stores by *Wholesome and Hearty*.

Makes 2 cups.
Serves 2.

Calories: 251 • Protein: (g) 9 • Carbs: (g) 9 • Fat: (g) 22 •
Sat. Fat: (g) 2 • Cholesterol: (mg) 0 • Fiber: (g) 5 • Sodium: (mg) 12

Strawberry Milk

1 cup Almond Milk
1/2 cup strawberries
1 tsp. sweetener

DIRECTIONS:
Blend until smooth.

Banana Milk

1 cup Almond Milk
1 banana

DIRECTIONS:
1. Blend in blender until smooth.
2. Add a little nutmeg and vanilla for a special flavor variation.

Apple Milk

1 cup fresh apple juice
1 banana
1 cup Almond Milk

DIRECTIONS:
Blend in blender until smooth.

Strawberry Shake

2 frozen bananas
1 cup fresh or frozen strawberries
1 cup Almond Milk
sweetener, if needed

DIRECTIONS:
Blend in blender until smooth.

Peach Shake

2 cups Almond Milk
2 frozen bananas
1 – 2 ripe peaches
Sprinkle of cinnamon

DIRECTIONS:
Blend in blender until smooth.

Banana Shake

2 cups Almond Milk
3 frozen bananas

DIRECTIONS:
Blend in blender until smooth.

Carob Chip Shake

2 cups Almond Milk
3 frozen bananas
1 Tbl. carob chips, sweetened or unsweetened

DIRECTIONS:
Blend in blender until smooth.

NOTE:
Substitution:
☆ Sunspire Chocolate Chips can be substituted for the carob chips. Sunspire chips are sweetened with barley malt instead of refined sugar.

Carob or Chocolate Syrup

A base for hot chocolate or great frostings.

1/2 cup milk (soy, rice, almond or, dairy)
1/2 cup carob powder — or cocoa powder
1/4 cup almond butter
1/4 – 1/2 cup maple syrup

DIRECTIONS:

Blend all ingredients in blender until smooth.
Keeps well in the refrigerator.

Makes 1 cup syrup.

Calories: 116 • Protein: (g) 4 • Carbs: (g) 7 • Fat: (g) 10 •
Sat. Fat: (g) 1 • Cholesterol: (mg) 0 • Fiber: (g) 3 • Sodium: (mg) 5

Hot Chocolate

Soothing drink from the aforementioned syrup.

1 cup milk (soy, rice, almond, or dairy)
2 – 3 Tbl. hot chocolate syrup

DIRECTIONS:

1. Place all ingredients in a small saucepan and heat to a simmer.
2. Pour into a mug and enjoy.

Makes 1 cup.

Calories: 194 • Protein: (g) 10 • Carbs: (g) 11 • Fat: (g) 15 •
Sat. Fat: (g) 2 • Cholesterol: (mg) 0 • Fiber: (g) 6 • Sodium: (mg) 35

Oat Milk

A soothing beverage for children.

1 cup whole oats
5 cups water
1 tsp. vanilla

DIRECTIONS:

1. Combine all ingredients in pan.
2. Bring to a boil, lower heat, cover and simmer 1 hour. Strain.

Makes approximately 1 cup.

Calories: 325 • Protein: (g) 13 • Carbs: (g) 54 • Fat: (g) 5 •
Sat. Fat: (g) 1 • Cholesterol: (mg) 0 • Fiber: (g) 9 • Sodium: (mg) 38

Rice (or Soy) Milk

Rice milk can be made easily and inexpensively at home. This is an adapted recipe from a Lifestyle for Health Newsletter reader.

1 cup sweet brown rice flour — or regular rice flour or soy flour
3 cups pure water

---

1 drop liquid lecithin
2 Tbl. olive oil — optional
1/2 tsp. vanilla — or to taste
1 Tbl. sweetener — or to taste
1/8 tsp. sea salt — or to taste

1/8 tsp. xanthan gum (found in health food stores)

DIRECTIONS:

1. To make **Rice (Soy) Base**, cook rice — or soy — flour and water in heavy metal pan (or double boiler) for 20 to 30 minutes, or until thickened.
2. Mix 1/3 cup **Rice (Soy) Base** and lecithin, olive oil, vanilla, sweetener, and sea salt in a blender.
3. Add 1 quart of water (do this in stages) along with xanthum gum (used to help emulsify) while blender is whipping. Add more rice base if too thin, more water if too thick.
4. Shake before using.
5. Refrigerate.

Makes 4 1/2 cups.

Per 1 cup:

Calories: 218 • Protein: (g) 3 • Carbs: (g) 34 • Fat: (g) 8 •
Sat. Fat: (g) 1 • Cholesterol: (mg) 0 • Fiber: (g) 2 • Sodium: (mg) 156

Cashew Cream

A thicker milk can be made from cashews. It has practically no saturated fat and no cholesterol. Since it is rich, it should be used in moderation.

1/2 cup of raw cashews
1 1/2 cups of water

---

2 tsp. sweetener (brown rice syrup or pure maple syrup)

DIRECTIONS:

1. Place cashews and enough water to cover blender blades in blender. Blend until creamy.
2. Add enough water and preferred sweetener to get the desired taste and consistency.

NOTES:

☆ This recipe multiplies well.

Variation:

☆ A variation of cashew cream can also be used to replace whipped cream. Use 1 cup raw cashews, 1 cup water. Blend this in a blender until smooth. Slowly, with blender running, add 1 cup of canola oil until cream thickens. Blend in 3 to 5 tablespoons of sweetener and approximately 1/2 teaspoon of vanilla to flavor the "cream." Chill the "cream" and it will stiffen. Refrigerate.

☆ Sunflower or sesame seeds can be substituted for cashews.

Makes 2 cups.

Per 1 cup:

Calories: 262 • Protein: (g) 7 • Carbs: (g) 18 • Fat: (g) 20 •
Sat. Fat: (g) 4 • Cholesterol: (mg) 0 • Fiber: (g) 1 • Sodium: (mg) 12

Notes:

Golden Grains

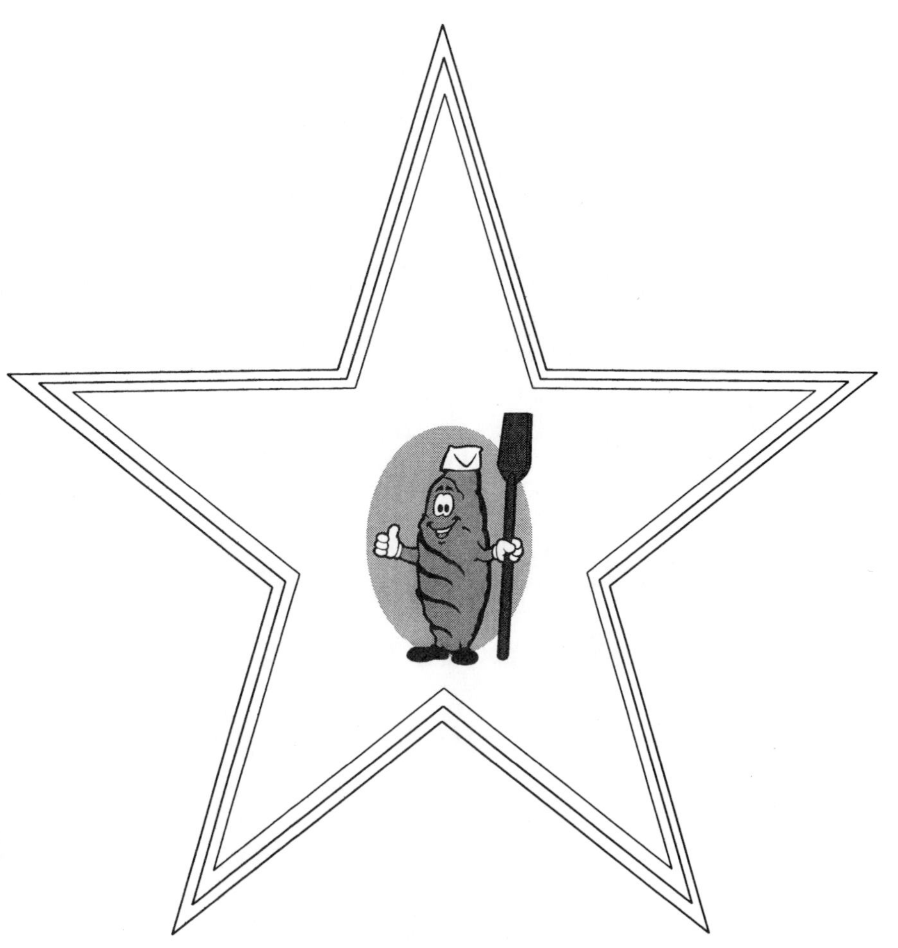

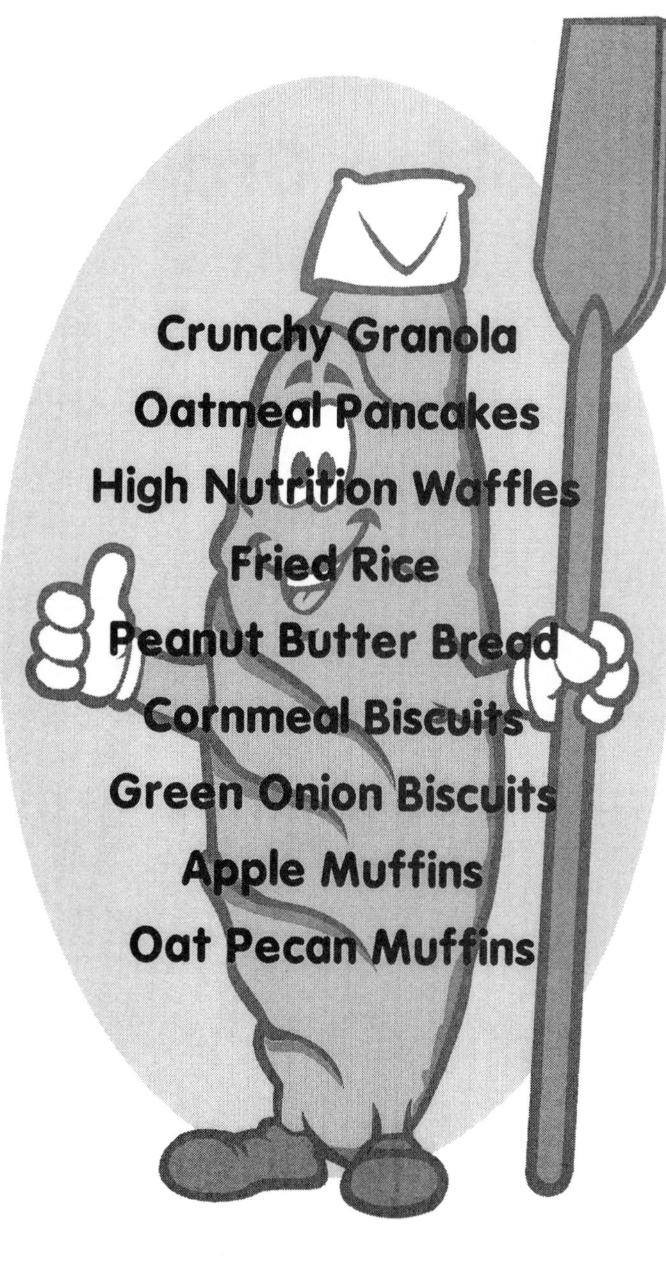

Crunchy Granola
Oatmeal Pancakes
High Nutrition Waffles
Fried Rice
Peanut Butter Bread
Cornmeal Biscuits
Green Onion Biscuits
Apple Muffins
Oat Pecan Muffins

Crunchy Granola

Add dried fruit when granola has cooled. This granola can also be added to muffins or coffee cakes for extra crunch.

2 cups rolled oats
1/2 cup barley flour – or whole wheat
2 Tbl. sunflower seeds
2 Tbl. chopped almonds
2 Tbl. chopped pecans
1/4 tsp. salt
1/2 tsp. ground cinnamon
1/4 tsp. ground nutmeg

1/4 cup maple syrup
1/4 cup canola oil
1 tsp. vanilla extract

DIRECTIONS:

1. Mix dry ingredients well.
2. Mix liquid ingredients and stir into the dry ingredients.
3. Spread on an oiled cookie sheet.
4. Bake at 325° for 20 – 45 minutes, stirring often (be careful not to let the granola burn). The amount of baking time is dependent upon depth of granola and size of baking sheet. Cool.
5. Add dried fruit (such as currants, raisins, or dried blueberries) after baking time.

NOTE:

☆ Store in refrigerator in an airtight container.

Makes 3 1/2 cups.

Calories: 253 • Protein: (g) 6 • Carbs: (g) 32 • Fat: (g) 16 •
Sat. Fat: (g) 5 • Cholesterol: (mg) 0 • Fiber: (g) 4 • Sodium: (mg) 100

Oatmeal Pancakes

Well worth a little time to make this on the weekend and freeze extras for during the week.

1 1/4 cups boiling water
1 1/4 cups milk (soy, rice, almond, or dairy)
2 cups rolled oats
2 Tbl. honey — or other sweetener

---

1 – 2 Tbl. oil
2 eggs — or substitute

---

1 cup barley flour — or whole wheat flour
2 tsp. baking powder
1/2 tsp. salt

DIRECTIONS:

1. Combine water, milk, oats, and honey in bowl. Cover and let set 30 – 45 minutes.
2. Stir in oil and eggs.
3. Stir dry ingredients together and add to the oat mixture. Let set a few minutes, if time permits.
4. Bake on hot, oiled griddle. Turn when top is bubbly.

NOTES:

Variations:

☆ Blueberry: add 1 – 2 cups blueberries to batter
☆ Apple: add 1 – 2 cups chopped apples to batter
☆ Banana: add 1 cup (2 ripe) mashed bananas to batter

Makes 16 – 20 4" pancakes.

Calories: 316 • Protein: (g) 13 • Carbs: (g) 48 • Fat: (g) 10 •
Sat. Fat: (g) 10 • Cholesterol: (mg) 86 • Fiber: (g) 6 • Sodium: (mg) 492

High Nutrition Waffles

These are hearty, crunchy, and freeze well.

1 3/4 cups spelt flour — or whole wheat
1 Tbl. baking powder
1/2 tsp. salt
1/3 cup wheat germ — or oat bran

---

2 eggs, separated — or only 3 egg whites
1/4 cup oil — or substitute
1 1/2 cups milk (soy, rice, almond, or dairy)

1/2 cup sunflower seeds
1/4 cup sesame seeds

DIRECTIONS:

1. Stir together the dry ingredients.
2. Mix the egg yolks and oil. Add the milk.
3. Stir into the dry ingredients along with the seeds.
4. Beat egg whites until stiff, but not dry, and fold into the batter.
5. Pour batter into center of hot prepared waffle iron. Bake about 5 minutes or until steaming stops. Remove carefully.
6. Serve with Honey Cinnamon Topping on page 268.

Makes 4 servings.

Calories: 603 • Protein: (g) 23 • Carbs: (g) 57 • Fat: (g) 37 •
Sat. Fat: (g) 6 • Cholesterol: (mg) 119 • Fiber: (g) 12 • Sodium: (mg) 698

Fried Rice

A great way to use cold brown rice. One of our weekly favorites.

1 onion, chopped
1 clove garlic, minced
1 Tbl. olive oil

---

1 10-oz. pkg. frozen peas

---

4 cups brown rice, cold, cooked
tamari, to taste

DIRECTIONS:

1. Sauté onion and garlic in oil.
2. Add peas and sauté until cooked.
3. Stir in rice and tamari and cook until done.

NOTES:

☆ Tamari is a superior soy sauce that is lower in sodium and better in flavor.

Variations:

☆ Add grated carrots, sliced mushrooms and/or bean sprouts for variety. Add as many vegetables as possible and this becomes a meal in itself.

Serves 6.

Calories: 208 • Protein: (g) 6 • Carbs: (g) 38 • Fat: (g) 3 •
Sat. Fat: (g) 1 • Cholesterol: (mg) 0 • Fiber: (g) 3 • Sodium: (mg) 374

Peanut Butter Bread

An easy to make muffin. Spread with a jam for an easy 'peanut butter and jelly sandwich.'

1/2 cup peanut butter — or almond butter
1/2 cup honey — or other sweetener
3 Tbl. oil
2 eggs — or substitute
1/2 cup carrot, grated
2 medium ripe bananas, mashed

1/4 cup milk (soy, rice, almond, or dairy)

1/4 tsp. cinnamon and nutmeg and allspice
1 tsp. vanilla
1/8 tsp. salt
1 tsp. baking powder
1 tsp. baking soda
1 3/4 cups spelt flour — or whole wheat

DIRECTIONS:

1. Blend the peanut butter, honey, oil, eggs, carrots, and bananas. Add the milk.
2. Mix the dry ingredients and add to the peanut butter mixture.
3. Bake at 300° in 3 well oiled mini-loaf pans for about 30 minutes or until done. Can be made in muffin pans.
4. Freeze extras.

Makes 1 large loaf or 2 – 3 mini-loaves.

Calories: 232 • Protein: (g) 6 • Carbs: (g) 33 • Fat: (g) 10 • Sat. Fat: (g) 2 • Cholesterol: (mg) 36 • Fiber: (g) 4 • Sodium: (mg) 210

Cornmeal Biscuits

A great biscuit. Make it large and use as a sandwich base. Make it smaller and serve with bean or lentil soup.

1/2 cup barley flour — or whole pastry
1 cup spelt flour — or whole wheat pastry
3/4 cup cornmeal
1/4 cup Sucanat — or granular sweetener
2 tsp. baking powder
1/4 tsp. salt

---

4 Tbl. butter — or oil

1/2 cup buttermilk, approximately

DIRECTIONS:

1. Mix all dry ingredients in a bowl.
2. Cut in butter.
3. Stir in buttermilk.
4. Drop by spoonfuls (or cut with biscuit cutter) onto oiled baking sheet (or use parchment paper) and bake at 400° for about 15 minutes or until done.

NOTE:

Substitutions:

☆ Buttermilk may be replaced with yogurt or 1/2 cup less 1/2 Tbl. milk (almond, rice, or soy) plus 1/2 Tbl. vinegar or lemon juice.

Makes 12 biscuits.

Calories: 126 • Protein: (g) 3 • Carbs: (g) 21 • Fat: (g) 4 • Sat. Fat: (g) 2 • Cholesterol: (mg) 11 • Fiber: (g) 3 • Sodium: (mg) 145

Green Onion Biscuits

An alternative to plain biscuits. These biscuits are great with soup. Make them larger and they are a great base for sandwiches.

1 cup barley flour — or whole wheat pastry
1 cup spelt flour — or whole wheat pastry
4 tsp. baking powder
1/4 tsp. salt
2 tsp. dry dill weed — optional
1/2 cup minced green onion

1/3 cup butter — or oil

3/4 cup buttermilk — or substitute

DIRECTIONS:

1. Mix all dry ingredients together.
2. Cut in butter or oil until blended to a coarse cornmeal texture.
3. Add enough buttermilk to form a ball. Do not overmix.
4. Drop by spoonfuls onto oiled baking sheet. (Or, knead slightly, roll out, cut into shapes, and bake.)
5. Bake at 400° for about 15 minutes or until done. The bottom should be golden brown.

Makes 10 – 12 medium size biscuits.

Calories: 225 • Protein: (g) 6 • Carbs: (g) 32 • Fat: (g) 11 •
Sat. Fat: (g) 6 • Cholesterol: (mg) 28 • Fiber: (g) 6 • Sodium: (mg) 459

Apple Muffins

A tasty muffin that is high in fiber and complex carbohydrates.

2 egg whites
3/4 cup milk (soy, almond, rice, or dairy)
1 medium apple, grated or chopped
1/2 cup currants
1/4 cup canola oil — or substitute
1/3 cup honey — or maple syrup

---

1 3/4 cups spelt flour — or whole wheat
1 Tbl. non-aluminum baking powder
1/2 tsp. cinnamon

DIRECTIONS:

1. Beat egg whites and stir in milk, apples, currants, oil, and honey.
2. Mix together dry ingredients.
3. Combine and stir briefly.
4. Fill oiled or lined muffin tin 2/3 – 3/4 full.
5. Bake at 400° for about 20 minutes.

Makes about 12 muffins.

Calories: 224 • Protein: (g) 5 • Carbs: (g) 38 • Fat: (g) 8 •
Sat. Fat: (g) 1 • Cholesterol: (mg) 3 • Fiber: (g) 5 • Sodium: (mg) 199

Oat Pecan Muffins

The best muffins I can prepare. They're a hit every time. Make extra and freeze.

1 cup barley flour — or whole wheat pastry
1/2 cup oats
1 1/4 tsp. baking powder
1/2 tsp. baking soda
1/2 tsp. cinnamon
1/4 tsp. nutmeg
1/4 tsp. salt

1/4 cup maple syrup
1 egg — or substitute
2 Tbl. oil
1/2 cup milk (soy, rice, almond, or dairy)
1 banana, mashed

---

2 – 4 Tbl. sesame seeds *and* sunflower seeds *and* chopped pecans

DIRECTIONS:

1. Mix all dry ingredients together.
2. Mix all liquid ingredients with the banana. Stir into the dry ingredients.
3. Stir in the seeds and nuts.
4. Pour into oiled or lined muffin tins. Bake at 400° for 15 minutes or until done.

NOTES:

☆ Recipe doubles and freezes well.

Substitutions:

☆ Banana may be replaced with 1 ripe peach, diced.

Makes 12 muffins.

Calories: 163 • Protein: (g) 5 • Carbs: (g) 19 • Fat: (g) 9 •
Sat. Fat: (g) 1 • Cholesterol: (mg) 19 • Fiber: (g) 2 • Sodium: (mg) 159

Notes:

Super Veggies

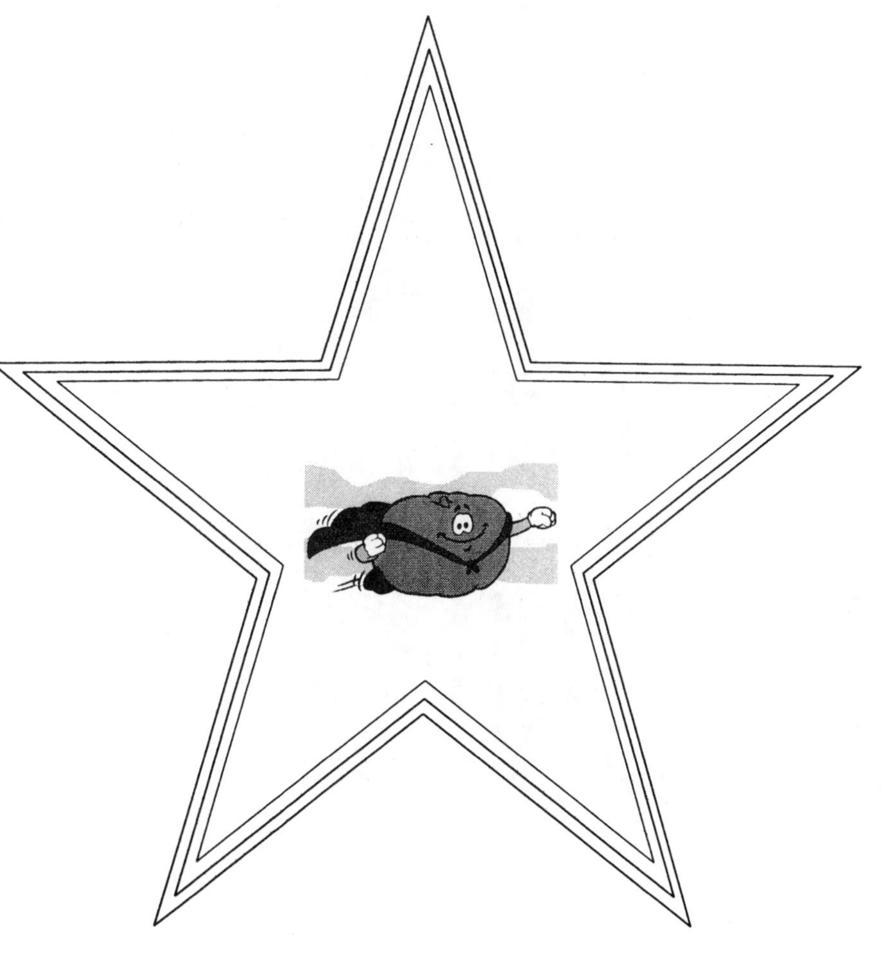

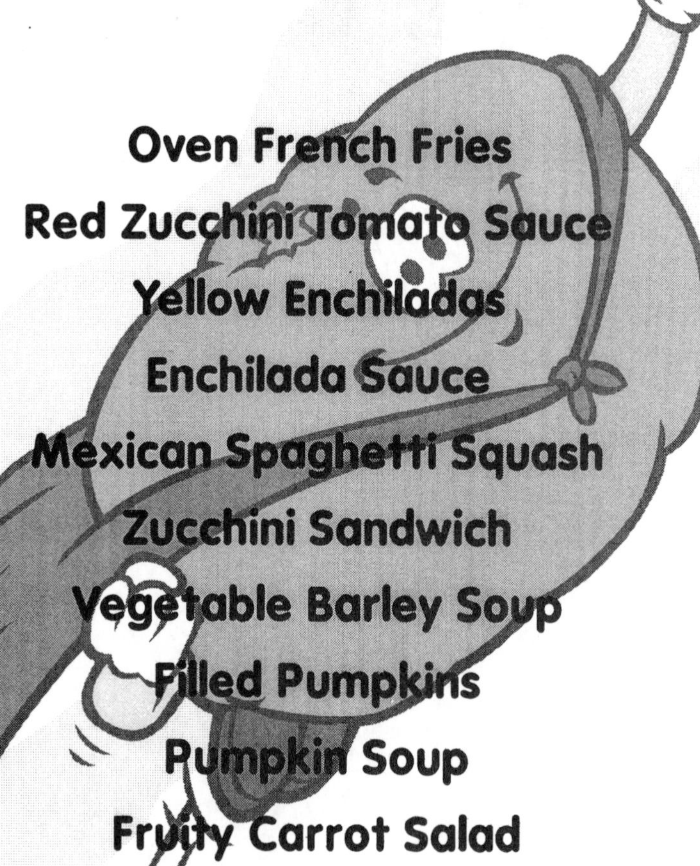

Oven French Fries

Red Zucchini Tomato Sauce

Yellow Enchiladas

Enchilada Sauce

Mexican Spaghetti Squash

Zucchini Sandwich

Vegetable Barley Soup

Filled Pumpkins

Pumpkin Soup

Fruity Carrot Salad

Oven French Fries

This has become a family favorite that is faster than a baked potato and uses less oil. Forest recently got me a little gadget that makes fast work out of making julienne strips from vegetables. So we have French Fries with the "right" shape.

Potatoes — use as many potatoes as necessary to make enough julienne strips to form a single layer of fries on an oiled cookie sheet.

DIRECTIONS:

1. Place the cut potatoes in a large bowl. Toss the potatoes with Spectrum Olive Oil (any good olive oil will work, this is my favorite).
2. Sprinkle potatoes with Parsley Patch Saltless Garlic Seasoning (another of my favorites). Toss with 2 forks. Spread out on an oiled cookie sheet.
3. Bake at 425°. Stir after 15 minutes. Keep baking until desired crispness is reached, about 20 minutes longer.
4. Serve alone or with Annie's Barbecue Sauce for a real taste sensation.

NOTE:

☆ The fewer the fries on the pan, the more crisp they will be. If there are too many layers of fries they will cook but not be very crispy.

Calories: 340 • Protein: (g) 7 • Carbs: (g) 78 • Fat: (g) 0 •
Sat. Fat: (g) 0 • Cholesterol: (mg) 0 • Fiber: (g) 2 • Sodium: (mg) 22

Red Zucchini Tomato Sauce

A tasty vegetable sauce to serve in place of regular pasta or tomato sauce.

2 – 3 zucchini, ends removed
1 onion
1 carrot, cleaned, ends removed
1/2 green or red bell pepper end and seeds removed
1 clove garlic, minced
1 large bay leaf
1/2 tsp. basil
1/4 tsp. marjoram
1/4 tsp. salt

---

1 tsp. olive oil — or stock
7 – 8 ripe tomatoes, stems removed and quartered

DIRECTIONS:

1. Place all vegetables except tomatoes in food processor and chop to medium texture (can be done by hand).
2. Sauté vegetables in oil. Add tomatoes and remaining ingredients. Cook for 20 minutes to 2 hours, depending on time and taste desired. Add water or stock, if too thick.

NOTE:

Substitution:

☆ Omit 1/2 of the zucchini and use 1/4 finely chopped eggplant.

Makes 3 cups.

Calories: 45 • Protein: (g) 2 • Carbs: (g) 9 • Fat: (g) 1 •
Sat. Fat: (g) 0 • Cholesterol: (mg) 0 • Fiber: (g) 3 • Sodium: (mg) 80

Yellow Enchiladas

By calling them enchiladas, most children will never notice that the filling is yellow or green squash.

1 large onion, chopped
2 cloves garlic, minced
1 tsp. olive oil

3/4 pound yellow summer or zucchini squash, chopped
1/2 of 4 oz. can chopped green chilies — optional
Sauce*

---

8 whole wheat or corn tortillas
garnishes

DIRECTIONS:

1. Sauté onion and garlic in oil. Add squash and simmer about 5 minutes. Drain. Stir in chilies and a third of the sauce.
2. Place about 1/4 – 1/3 cup filling into tortilla and roll up.
3. Place in 12" x 7" oiled pan. Cover with remaining sauce. Bake, covered, at 400° for about 30 minutes.
4. Garnish as desired with fresh chopped tomatoes or salsa, lettuce and avocado.

NOTE:

* Sauce recipe is found on next page.

Serves 3 – 4.

Calories: 37 • Protein: (g) 2 • Carbs: (g) 6 • Fat: (g) 1 •
Sat. Fat: (g) 0 • Cholesterol: (mg) 0 • Fiber: (g) 2 • Sodium: (mg) 239

* Enchilada Sauce

This sauce is excellent so you may want to make an extra batch.

1 Tbl. olive oil
2 Tbl. rice flour — or whole wheat flour

---

1 tsp. chili powder — or Frontier Mexican Seasoning
1/4 tsp. salt — or tamari
pinch cayenne pepper
1 – 2 Tbl. chopped chilies
1 cup milk (soy, rice, or almond)

3/4 cup shredded cheese

DIRECTIONS:

1. Heat oil and stir in flour.
2. Add remaining ingredients and stir until bubbly.
3. Stir in cheese.

NOTE:

Substitution:

☆ Cheese may be replaced with a raw milk, low fat, or Monterey Jack cheese.

Makes approximately 2 cups.

Calories: 113 • Protein: (g) 5 • Carbs: (g) 6 • Fat: (g) 8 •
Sat. Fat: (g) 3 • Cholesterol: (mg) 9 • Fiber: (g) 2 • Sodium: (mg) 220

Mexican Spaghetti Squash

A crunchy, southwestern style of serving spaghetti squash. If your family is not ready for the spaghetti squash, use all pasta spaghetti, or half spaghetti and half squash.

1 – 3 pounds spaghetti squash

1/4 cup onion, chopped — or scallion, chopped
1 clove garlic, minced
1 tsp. olive oil

1/2 cup sweet red pepper, chopped
1/2 cup green pepper, chopped
1/2 cup corn
1/4 cup chicken stock — or vegetable stock
4 Tbl. parsley, minced
1 Tbl. cider vinegar
1/4 tsp. salt — or tamari
1/4 – 1/2 tsp. Frontier Mexican Seasoning — or cumin

1/2 cup black olives, sliced — optional
1/4 cup jicama, chopped — or nuts

DIRECTIONS:

1. Halve squash, discard seeds. Place cut side down in a large oiled baking dish. Add 1/2" water, cover and bake at 350° for about 30 – 45 minutes or until done (sides will pierce easily with a knife or fork).
2. While squash is cooking, sauté onion and garlic in oil. Add remaining ingredients except the olives and jicama. Cook until tender.
3. Use a fork to shred and separate the squash pulp into strands, reserving shells. In a bowl, toss the squash pulp, vegetable mixture, olives, and jicama. Transfer back to the squash shells.

Makes 6 – 8 servings.

Calories: 74 • Protein: (g) 2 • Carbs: (g) 13 • Fat: (g) 3 •
Sat. Fat: (g) 0 • Cholesterol: (mg) 0 • Fiber: (g) 2 • Sodium: (mg) 213

Zucchini Sandwich

A delicious and easy sandwich that even pleases "zucchini haters." Be sure to try it and the variations.

1 Tbl. olive oil
1/2 onion, chopped
1 clove garlic, minced

1/2 tsp. basil
1/4 tsp. oregano
1/2 tsp. thyme

---

2 cups zucchini, sliced — or chopped
2 Tbl. carrots, grated

---

hamburger buns, spelt, split
fresh tomato, thinly sliced
Parmesan cheese

DIRECTIONS:

1. Sauté the onion and garlic in oil. Add herbs and sauté until the onion is tender. Add the zucchini and carrot and sauté.
2. Cover a hamburger bun half with the zucchini mixture. Place a tomato slice on top and sprinkle with Parmesan.
3. Broil until Parmesan is melted.

NOTES:

☆ Use only a good Parmesan cheese, no fake cheese, please.

Substitutions:

☆ Spelt hamburger buns may be replaced with whole grain bun/bread.

☆ Parmesan cheese may be replaced with Brewers's yeast.

Variation:

☆ Spread some pizza sauce over the bun before adding the zucchini mixture. The tomato slice may be used or omitted.

Makes 6 – 8.

Calories: 169 • Protein: (g) 7 • Carbs: (g) 26 • Fat: (g) 5 •
Sat. Fat: (g) 1 • Cholesterol: (mg) 2 • Fiber: (g) 3 • Sodium: (mg) 291

Vegetable Barley Soup

A very satisfying and nutritious soup. This is wonderful with a chunk of homemade bread on a cold winter night in front of a roaring fire.

8 cups chicken stock — or strong vegetable stock
1 16 oz. can tomatoes, undrained
1 onion, chopped
1 cup carrots, chopped
1 cup celery, chopped
1 cup broccoli, chopped
1 cup peas
1 cup potatoes, chopped — optional
2/3 cup barley
1/3 cup green pepper, chopped
1 Tbl. fresh basil, torn — or 1 tsp. dried basil
1 Tbl. fresh thyme, torn — or 1 tsp. dried thyme
1 tsp. tamari — or sea salt
2 bay leaves

DIRECTIONS:

1. Heat stock and add remaining ingredients. Cook for 1 hour or all day in a crockpot.
2. Remove bay leaves to serve.

May be made in advance and refrigerated or frozen.

Serves 6 – 8.

Calories: 170 • Protein: (g) 10 • Carbs: (g) 29 • Fat: (g) 2 •
Sat. Fat: (g) 0 • Cholesterol: (mg) 0 • Fiber: (g) 5 • Sodium: (mg) 187

Filled Pumpkins

Mini pumpkins become a truly fun food to stuff and have children help in the preparation. It's like decorating pumpkins. Save the seeds and roast them as in the following recipe.

6 – 8 pumpkins, cleaned

---

3 pounds fresh spinach, cleaned, stems removed

---

1 small onion, chopped
1 clove garlic, minced
1 Tbl. olive oil
4 Tbl. rice flour
2 cups hot water — or stock
1/2 tsp. tamari — or sea salt
1 Tbl. light miso — optional
1/2 tsp. nutmeg

DIRECTIONS:

1. Remove the 'lid' from the pumpkin. Remove the seeds and stringy flesh. Rinse well.
2. Place pumpkin upside down in pan with 1/2" of water, cover and bake at 350° for about 45 minutes, or until done.
3. Steam spinach. Cool, squeeze out water, and chop.
4. Sauté onion and garlic in oil until transparent. Stir in flour until blended. Add water slowly, stirring until smooth. Bring to a boil and add seasonings. Cook about 5 minutes. Adjust seasoning, as needed.
5. Stir in cooked spinach. Place in cooked pumpkin and set the 'lids' on at an angle. Reheat, if needed.

NOTE:

Substitution:

☆ Spinach may be replaced with either swiss chard or broccoli or a combination.

Serves 6 – 8.

Calories: 387 • Protein: (g) 10 • Carbs: (g) 77 • Fat: (g) 5 •
Sat. Fat: (g) 1 • Cholesterol: (mg) 0 • Fiber: (g) 8 • Sodium: (mg) 187

Pumpkin Soup

Another way to use fresh or canned pumpkin. Leftover, cooked sweet potatoes or yams can also be used. Serve this in a large pumpkin for more visual appeal.

1 tsp. olive oil
4 green onions, minced
1/2 pound mushrooms, sliced
2 – 3 tsp. curry powder

---

2 cups pumpkin, cooked — or canned
4 cups chicken broth — or vegetable stock
1 cup water
1 cup milk (soy, rice, or almond)
sea salt — or tamari
parsley

DIRECTIONS:

1. Sauté onions and mushrooms in oil. Stir in curry powder and stir well.
2. Stir in pumpkin, broth, and water and simmer, covered, for about 15 minutes.
3. Slowly stir in milk and desired sea salt or tamari.
4. Garnish with fresh parsley.

Serves 4 – 6.

Calories: 128 • Protein: (g) 8 • Carbs: (g) 8 • Fat: (g) 3 •
Sat. Fat: (g) 1 • Cholesterol: (mg) 0 • Fiber: (g) 5 • Sodium: (mg) 16

Fruity Carrot Salad

An easy salad kids can make for themselves.

1 pound carrots, grated
1 8 oz. can pineapple chunks
1/2 cup currants — or raisins

1/2 cup orange juice — or pineapple juice
1/4 cup plain low-fat yogurt, optional

DIRECTIONS:

1. Combine carrots, pineapple, and currants.
2. Blend juice and yogurt in blender until smooth.
3. Pour over the carrots.

Serves 4.

Calories: 123 • Protein: (g) 3 • Carbs: (g) 29 • Fat: (g) 0 •
Sat. Fat: (g) 0 • Cholesterol: (mg) 0 • Fiber: (g) 5 • Sodium: (mg) 55

Yummy-For-Your-Tummy Main Dishes

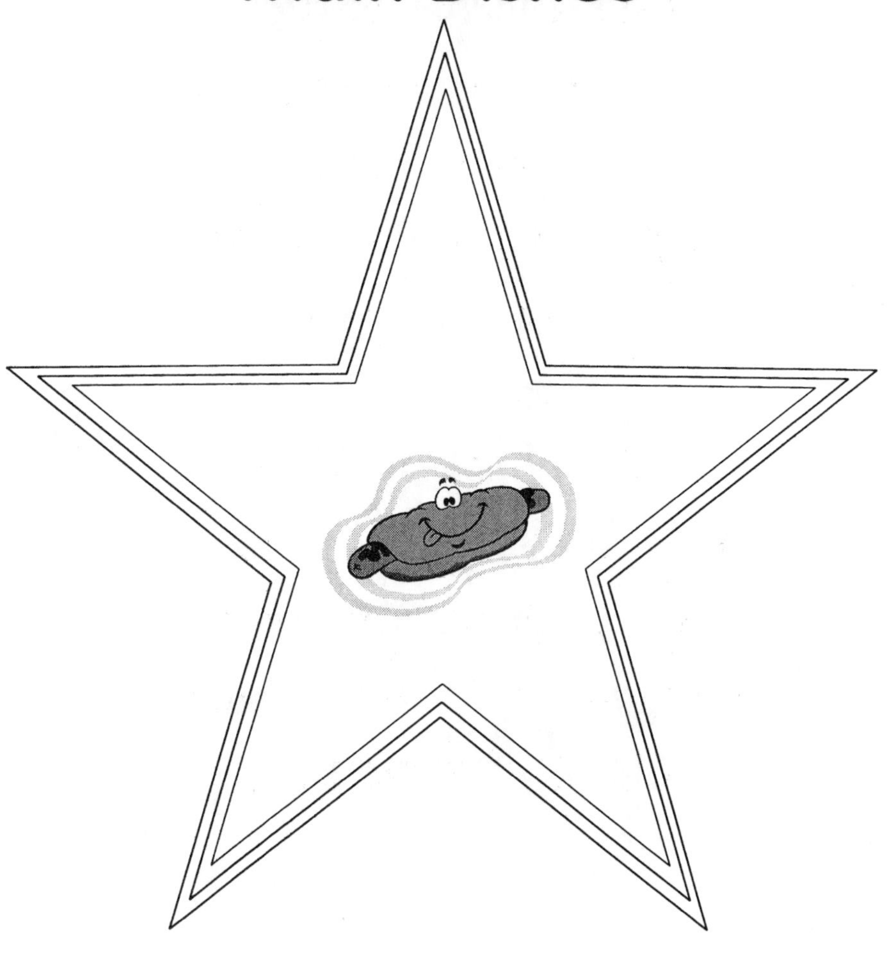

Kid's Zucchini Lasagna

Yummy Pizza

Pizza Crust

Refried Beans Burritos

Burrito Cups

Terrific Franks

Cornmeal Baking Mix

Honeyed Sesame "Chicken"

Crispy Fried "Chicken"

Spaghetti with "Meatballs"

Chunky Potato Soup

Kid's Zucchini Lasagna

A healthy version of lasagna that substitutes zucchini for the noodles. Kids really like this one. Check out the vegetarian option.

1 pound ground turkey
1 onion, chopped
2 cloves garlic, minced
2 cups pasta sauce
1 1/2 cups cottage cheese — or substitute
1 egg, beaten — or substitute
4 medium zucchini
1/2 cup mozzarella cheese — or soy
1/3 cup Parmesan cheese — or soy

DIRECTIONS:

1. Brown the turkey, onion, and garlic. Drain off all fat. Stir in pasta sauce. Simmer for about 10 minutes.
2. Combine the cottage cheese and egg.
3. Slice the zucchini lengthwise into 1/8" thick slices.
4. Place half of zucchini into oiled 13" x 9" pan. Top with half of cottage cheese mixture and half of the sauce mixture. Repeat layers.
5. Sprinkle top with mozzarella and Parmesan cheese.
6. Bake uncovered at 350° for 1 hour.
7. Let stand 10 – 15 minutes before slicing.

NOTES:

Substitutions:

☆ 1 pound ground turkey may be replaced with crumbled tempeh.

☆ Pasta sauce may be replaced with 2 cups tomato sauce with 1 tsp. basil, 1 tsp. oregano, 1/2 tsp. thyme, and 1/2 tsp. marjoram added.

☆ Cottage or ricotta cheese and egg may be replaced with the following, blended in a blender, until well blended:

1 pkg. Mori Nu "lite" Tofu, Firm	1/4 cup olive oil
1/4 tsp. salt	1/4 tsp. nutmeg

Serves 6.

Calories: 264 • Protein: (g) 29 • Carbs: (g) 14 • Fat: (g) 11 •
Sat. Fat: (g) 4 • Cholesterol: (mg) 102 • Fiber: (g) 4 • Sodium: (mg) 682

Yummy Pizza

A quick pizza with extra veggies. MY daughter calls it "the BEST pizza she ever ate."

1 pizza crust
1 jar pizza sauce
fresh spinach, chopped
sliced mushrooms
slivered red peppers
chopped sun dried tomatoes
sliced onions
organic, low-fat mozzarella cheese, sliced

DIRECTIONS:

1. Prebake the pizza crust at 425° for about 4 – 5 minutes, preferably on a pizza stone dusted with cornmeal.
2. Cover the pizza crust with the sauce. Place a layer of chopped spinach on top. Sprinkle with the remaining veggies. Place mozzarella cheese on top.
3. Bake an additional 5 – 10 minutes, or until done.

NOTES:

Substitutions:

☆ Pizza crust may be replaced with any purchased whole grain pizza crust. The crust on the next page is excellent.

☆ I prefer Muir or Enrico brand of pizza sauce. An excellent pizza sauce is in the *Lifestyle for Health* cookbook.

☆ Organic, low-fat mozzarella cheese may be replaced with any low-fat or tofu mozzarella cheese.

Serves 3 – 4.

Calories: 324 • Protein: (g) 15 • Carbs: (g) 57 • Fat: (g) 7 •
Sat. Fat: (g) 19 • Cholesterol: (mg) 7 • Fiber: (g) 2 • Sodium: (mg) 424

Pizza Crust

An excellent and easy alternative to "store-bought" crust.

1 1/2 – 2 cups spelt flour — or kamut
1 Tbl. olive oil
1/2 tsp. salt

---

2 tsp. yeast
3/4 cup water, approximately

DIRECTIONS:

1. Mix salt, flour, and olive oil together until crumbly.
2. Dissolve yeast in small amount of water, let proof about 4 minutes.
3. Add yeast and enough water to form a stiff ball. Knead for a few minutes until smooth. Let rise about 30 minutes.
4. Roll out on hot pizza stone sprinkled with cornmeal.
5. Bake as directed in step 1 of Pizza recipe on previous page.

NOTES:

☆ If using a Universal Bosch, make 4 – 6 times the recipe using the water-flour method, until dough cleans side of bowl.

☆ Partially baked crusts freeze very well. Remove from freezer and proceed as usual.

Makes 1 large or 4 individual crusts.

Calories: 236 • Protein: (g) 9 • Carbs: (g) 49 • Fat: (g) 4 •
Sat. Fat: (g) 0 • Cholesterol: (mg) 0 • Fiber: (g) 11 • Sodium: (mg) 300

Refried Bean Burritos

A great way to use pinto beans, black beans, or even lentils. Use in all sorts of ways. Make a large batch and freeze in small quantities.

1 pound of dry beans, cooked*
1 tsp. olive oil
1 onion, chopped
1 – 2 cloves garlic, minced
1/2 tsp. cumin
1/4 tsp. Caribe red pepper flakes
2 – 3 tsp. Frontier Mexican spice — or chili powder, to taste
1 pkg. tortillas

DIRECTIONS:

1. Sauté the onion and garlic in oil until translucent. Add spices and blend well.
2. Add mashed, cooked beans and stir until well blended. Simmer for about 10 – 15 minutes, or until desired consistency is reached.
3. To serve, roll in tortillas (whole wheat or corn) and serve as burritos. Or place in a taco shell (soft or hard) in place of the meat. Add lots of chopped lettuce (no iceberg, please), chopped tomatoes, salsa, and a low-fat cheese or tofu cheese.

NOTES:

Substitution:

☆ Two cans of refried beans may replace the one pound of raw beans.

* To cook beans:

Soak beans overnight in 6 cups water. Pour out water. Add enough water to cover and no salt (salt toughens beans and prevents them from becoming soft). A strip of kombu may be added to decrease flatulence, increase digestibility, and increase mineral content. Cook until beans are done. This can be done in a crockpot and cooked all day.

Serves 4 – 6.

Calories: 376 • Protein: (g) 13 • Carbs: (g) 64 • Fat: (g) 9 •
Sat. Fat: (g) 1 • Cholesterol: (mg) 0 • Fiber: (g) 8 • Sodium: (mg) 786

Burrito Cups

A great way to use homemade or purchased refried beans or lentils. Kids like the variety. The beans, meat, and tortillas are not a good food combination. All meat or all refried beans are a better combination with the tortillas.

6 – 8 whole wheat tortillas — or corn tortillas
2 Tbl. canola oil
1 Tbl. chili powder
1 pound ground organic turkey — or crumbled tempeh
1 cup refried beans
4 oz. soy cheese, grated
taco seasoning*
garnishes

DIRECTIONS:

1. Place tortilla in pan to soften or place in a steaming rack and steam until soft.
2. Brush tortilla with a little oil and place in an oiled custard cup.
3. Bake in 350° oven until crisp.
4. Brown ground turkey and drain off fat.
5. Mix in the taco seasoning mix* along with 1 Tbl. healthy catsup and 1/2 cup water. Simmer about 10 minutes.
6. Fill cups with meat, beans, and cheese. Broil until cheese melts.
7. Serve with garnishes (i.e., chopped lettuce, tomatoes, and salsa).

NOTE:

*Taco Seasoning Mix:

1 Tbl. instant minced onion
2 tsp. cumin
1/4 tsp. red pepper flakes
1/2 tsp. arrowroot
1 1/2 tsp. chili powder
1/2 tsp. sea salt
1/2 tsp. instant minced garlic
1/4 tsp. oregano

Mix all ingredients together.

Serves 4 – 6.

Calories: 517 • Protein: (g) 32 • Carbs: (g) 49 • Fat: (g) 23 •
Sat. Fat: (g) 3 • Cholesterol: (mg) 68 • Fiber: (g) 5 • Sodium: (mg) 1513

Terrific Franks

These treats make great snacks or quick and easy meals when combined with the suggested menu ideas. The tofu hot dogs make this a better food combining dish.

- 4 hot dogs, each cut into sixths and steamed
- 1 batch of cornbread batter (see recipe on next page)
- 2 Tbl. sesame seeds

DIRECTIONS:

1. Preheat oven to 400°.
2. Fill lined muffin tins one-half full of cornmeal batter. Place one hot dog piece on batter. Place a dollop of cornmeal batter on top. Sprinkle with sesame seeds.
3. Bake about 20 minutes or until done.

NOTES:

Substitutions:

☆ Hot dogs may be replaced with any of the many excellent tofu, turkey, and chicken hot dogs that are available.

☆ Use the cornbread baking mix on the following page or a prepared mix. There are several cornbread baking mixes on the market. Read the label to find one with whole grain flours.

Makes 12 muffins.

Calories: 427 • Protein: (g) 14 • Carbs: (g) 57 • Fat: (g) 18 •
Sat. Fat: (g) 4 • Cholesterol: (mg) 66 • Fiber: (g) 3 • Sodium: (mg) 1033

Cornmeal Baking Mix

The following is a mix from the Cornbread found in Lifestyle for Health cookbook.

1 1/2 cups cornmeal
1/2 cup barley flour — or whole wheat or quinoa flour
1 Tbl. baking powder
3/4 tsp. salt

---

1 egg — or substitute
1 cup milk — or substitute
1/4 cup honey
1 Tbl. canola oil

DIRECTIONS:

1. Mix dry ingredients.
2. Mix liquid ingredients. Add to dry mixture, until well blended.
3. If making Terrific Franks, proceed with directions, step 2 of that recipe.
4. If making cornbread, pour into oiled 9" x 9" pan. Bake at 350° for 30 – 35 minutes or until done.

NOTE:

Substitution:

☆ Rice Milk may be replaced with almond, soy, or low-fat milk.

Calories: 155 • Protein: (g) 3 • Carbs: (g) 25 • Fat: (g) 5 •
Sat. Fat: (g) 1 • Cholesterol: (mg) 27 • Fiber: (g) 2 • Sodium: (mg) 372

Honeyed Sesame "Chicken"

A favorite of young and old alike.

1/2 cup apple juice
3 Tbl. honey
3 Tbl. tamari
1/2 Tbl. lemon juice
2 Tbl. arrowroot powder
1 – 2 clove garlic, minced
1 1/4 tsp. fresh grated ginger root
1/4 – 1/2 tsp. Picante red pepper flakes
1/4 cup unhulled sesame seeds

1/2 – 1 pound natural chicken breast

DIRECTIONS:

1. Combine all ingredients except chicken in jar and shake to combine well.
2. Dip chicken in sesame mixture.
3. Sauté or stir fry chicken until done. Stir in any extra sauce and cook until thick.

NOTE:

Substitutions:

☆ Arrowroot powder may be replaced with corn starch.
☆ Fresh ginger root may be replaced with 1/4 to 1/2 tsp. dried ginger.
☆ Extra firm tofu could replace chicken for a vegetarian version of this recipe.

Serves 3.

Calories: 221 • Protein: (g) 9 • Carbs: (g) 33 • Fat: (g) 7 •
Sat. Fat: (g) 1 • Cholesterol: (mg) 12 • Fiber: (g) 2 • Sodium: (mg) 1021

Crispy Fried "Chicken"

A great dish that is lower in fat than traditional fried chicken.

1/3 cup low-fat yogurt
2 Tbl. lemon juice
2 tsp. fresh ginger, minced, peeled — or 1/2 tsp. dried ginger
1 clove garlic, minced
1/2 tsp. cumin
1/2 tsp. red pepper flakes

---

4 organic boned chicken breast halves, skinned
1 1/4 cups oat bran flake cereal, crushed

DIRECTIONS:

1. Combine all ingredients in bowl except chicken and cereal.
2. Add chicken to mixture, coating well. Cover and refrigerate overnight or for at least 4 hours.
3. Keeping marinade on chicken, coat chicken in crushed cereal.
4. Place on oiled baking sheet. Bake at 400° for about 50 minutes or until done.

NOTE:

Substitution:

☆ Replace chicken with chicken-flavored seitan for a tasty vegetarian option.

Serves 4.

Calories: 339 • Protein: (g) 57 • Carbs: (g) 10 • Fat: (g) 7 •
Sat. Fat: (g) 2 • Cholesterol: (mg) 147 • Fiber: (g) 2 • Sodium: (mg) 161

Spaghetti with "Meatballs"

A real twist on the old familiar meatballs. This adds complex carbohydrates, less fat, and is a better food combination than the traditional meatballs.

2 cups cooked grains*
3/4 cup mashed potatoes
1/4 cup grated Parmesan
1 onion, chopped
2 cloves garlic, minced
1/2 cup parsley, minced
1 tsp. Italian seasoning
1 tsp. tamari
1/2 tsp. thyme
1/2 tsp. red pepper flakes

1/4 cup olive oil
1 pound whole grain spaghetti, cooked
3 – 4 cups pasta sauce, hot

DIRECTIONS:

1. Combine all ingredients except oil, pasta, and sauce. Mix well and chill at least 30 minutes. Shape into 1" balls.
2. Place on oiled baking sheet and brush with oil. Bake at 400° for about 25 minutes, turning as needed to ensure even browning.
3. Combine meatballs with hot sauce. Pour over spaghetti.

NOTE:

* Cooked grains — cooked quinoa, amaranth, rice, or millet are good options. These are excellent grains to add to your diet. They are higher in protein than wheat, very tasty, and quick cooking. The *Lifestyle for Health* cookbook has a chapter on how to cook all kinds of grains.

Serves 4.

Calories: 650 • Protein: (g) 27 • Carbs: (g) 132 • Fat: (g) 6 •
Sat. Fat: (g) 2 • Cholesterol: (mg) 4 • Fiber: (g) 7 • Sodium: (mg) 1608

Chunky Potato Soup

It's delicious and sooooo easy. Try some today.

4 – 6 Tbl. rice flour — or whole wheat
2 Tbl. oil — or stock
4 – 6 cups rice milk — or soy, almond, or dairy
1 heaping Tbl. miso

---

4 cups diced potatoes
1 – 2 cups chopped broccoli florets
1/4 cup chopped, dried onion
1 Tbl. pesto — optional
1/2 tsp. basil
salt, to taste

DIRECTIONS:

1. Heat oil or stock.
2. Stir in flour until smooth. Add milk and miso slowly, stirring until smooth.
3. Stir in veggies and seasonings.
4. Let simmer until potatoes are tender.

Can be made in a crockpot: cook on low for 8 hours.

Serves 4.

Calories: 1100 • Protein: (g) 28 • Carbs: (g) 202 • Fat: (g) 21 •
Sat. Fat: (g) 3 • Cholesterol: (mg) 0 • Fiber: (g) 17 • Sodium: (mg) 247

Notes:

Best-For-Last Desserts

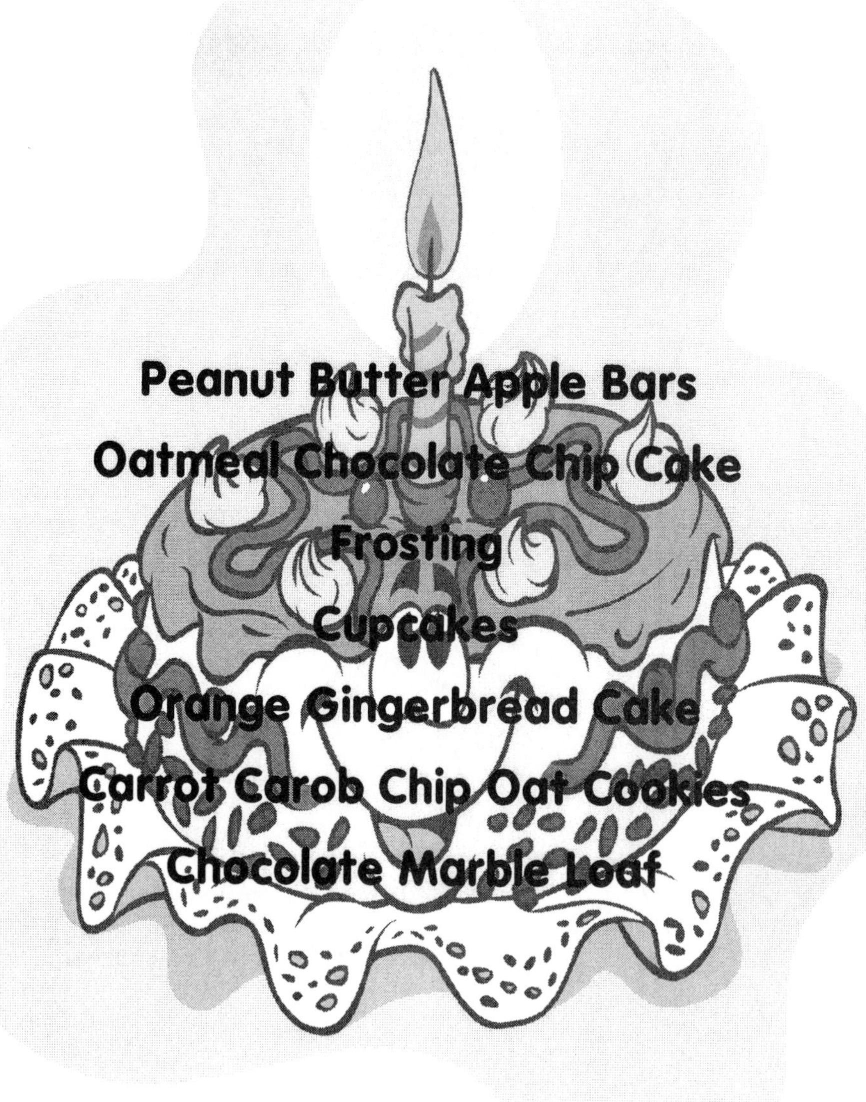

Peanut Butter Apple Bars

Oatmeal Chocolate Chip Cake

Frosting

Cupcakes

Orange Gingerbread Cake

Carrot Carob Chip Oat Cookies

Chocolate Marble Loaf

Peanut Butter Apple Bars

Although these are almost a cookie, they are quite similar to a "peanut butter and jelly sandwich" when split in half and spread with jam.

3/4 cup spelt flour — or whole wheat pastry
1/2 tsp. baking soda

3/4 cup peanut butter — or almond butter
1/2 cup oil — or substitute*
1/2 cup honey
1 tsp. vanilla
2 eggs — or egg substitute*

1/2 cup applesauce
1 1/4 cups oats
1/4 cup wheat germ — or oat bran

DIRECTIONS:

1. Mix spelt flour and baking soda.
2. In food processor, mix peanut butter, oil, honey, vanilla, and eggs. Stir in the applesauce. Add the flour mixture. Stir in the oats and wheat germ.
3. Place in oiled 9" x 13" pan. Bake at 350° about 25 minutes or until done.

NOTE:

* See substitutes in Appendix D.

Makes about 24 to 32 bars.

Calories: 166 • Protein: (g) 5 • Carbs: (g) 17 • Fat: (g) 10 •
Sat. Fat: (g) 1 • Cholesterol: (mg) 18 • Fiber: (g) 1 • Sodium: (mg) 34

Oatmeal Chocolate Chip Cake

A delicious cake that is as easy as any dump cake. It is excellent without any frosting.

1 3/4 cups boiling water
1 cup rolled oats

---

1 1/3 cups honey — or granular sweetener
1/2 cup oil — or substitute
2 eggs — or substitute

---

2 cups spelt flour — or whole wheat pastry flour
1 tsp. baking soda
1/2 tsp. salt
1 Tbl. cocoa or carob powder

---

1 cup Sunspire chocolate — or carob chips
1/2 cup chopped pecans — optional

DIRECTIONS:

1. Pour boiling water over oats. Let stand at room temperature for about 10 – 30 minutes.
2. Add honey and oil. Beat in eggs.
3. Combine all dry ingredients and mix into oat mixture.
4. Pour batter into an oiled 9" x 13" pan. Sprinkle pecans and chips on the top. Bake at 350° for about 30 – 40 minutes or until done.

Makes 20 squares.

Calories: 255 • Protein: (g) 4 • Carbs: (g) 39 • Fat: (g) 11 •
Sat. Fat: (g) 2 • Cholesterol: (mg) 23 • Fiber: (g) 2 • Sodium: (mg) 131

Frosting

An easy frosting that has no unrefined sugar and is easy to make.

1/4 cup milk (soy, rice, almond, or dairy)
1/4 cup cocoa — or carob powder
2 Tbl. almond butter
4 Tbl. maple syrup

---

4 tsp. arrowroot powder
1/4 cup milk (soy, rice, almond, or dairy)

DIRECTIONS:

1. Combine the first four ingredients to blender and blend until smooth. Transfer to a small pan.
2. Stir in arrowroot and remaining milk. Heat on low, stirring occasionally until it thickens. It will thicken more as it cools.

Makes 2 cups, enough for top of a 9" x 13" cake.

Calories: 17 • Protein: (g) 1 • Carbs: (g) 2 • Fat: (g) 1 •
Sat. Fat: (g) 0 • Cholesterol: (mg) 0 • Fiber: (g) 1 • Sodium: (mg) 1

Cupcakes

An easy "white" cupcake alternative for birthdays or special treats.

1 1/4 cups spelt flour — or whole wheat pastry flour
1 cup barley flour — or whole wheat pastry flour
1 Tbl. baking powder
1/4 tsp. sea salt

----

1 tsp. vanilla
1/2 cup canola oil — or oil substitute
1 cup milk (soy, rice, almond, or dairy)
1/2 cup maple syrup — or granular sweetener
2 eggs — or substitute

DIRECTIONS:

1. Mix all dry ingredients together.
2. Combine wet ingredients. Combine with dry ingredients and mix well.
3. Spoon into oiled or lined muffin tins about 2/3 full. Bake for 25 minutes at 375° or until done.

Can be frosted with frosting on previous page.

Makes about 12 cupcakes.

Calories: 168 • Protein: (g) 4 • Carbs: (g) 2 • Fat: (g) 11 •
Sat. Fat: (g) 1 • Cholesterol: (mg) 36 • Fiber: (g) 3 • Sodium: (mg) 185

Orange Gingerbread Cake

A nice change from chocolate, carob, or white cakes.

1 1/2 cups spelt four — or whole wheat pastry flour
1 cup barley flour — or whole wheat pastry flour
1 tsp. baking soda
1 tsp. baking powder
1/2 tsp. ginger
1/2 tsp. cloves
1/4 tsp. salt — optional

1/2 to 1 cup dates, chopped

---

2 egg whites
1/4 cup oil
1/2 cup orange juice — or water
1/2 cup milk (soy, rice, almond, or dairy)
1 cup maple syrup — or granular sweetener

DIRECTIONS:

1. Mix all dry ingredients together. Add dates and mix.
2. Beat egg whites, oil, juice, milk, and syrup well. Stir into flour mixture.
3. Pour into an oiled 9" x 13" pan and bake at 350° about 30 to 40 minutes or until done.

Makes 20 squares.

Calories: 92 • Protein: (g) 2 • Carbs: (g) 16 • Fat: (g) 3 • Sat. Fat: (g) 0 • Cholesterol: (mg) 0 • Fiber: (g) 3 • Sodium: (mg) 124

Carrot Carob Chip Oat Cookies

A quick cookie loaded with whole grain and complex carbohydrates.

1/2 cup peanut — or almond butter
1/3 cup honey
1/4 cup maple syrup
2 egg whites
1/4 cup water — or apple juice

---

1 cup spelt flour — or whole wheat pastry
1 cup grated carrots
1 cup rolled oats
1/2 tsp. baking powder
1/2 tsp. baking soda
1/4 tsp. nutmeg
1/4 tsp. cinnamon
1/4 tsp. salt

1/2 – 3/4 cup Sunspire carob chips

DIRECTIONS:

1. In food processor, mix peanut butter, honey, maple syrup, egg whites and water.
2. Mix all other ingredients except chips.
3. Stir in chips.
4. Drop by heaping teaspoonfuls onto oiled baking sheet. Bake at 375° for about 12 to 15 minutes or until done. (If cookie dough is too thin, add more oats.)

Makes 2 – 3 dozen.

Calories: 231 • Protein: (g) 7 • Carbs: (g) 34 • Fat: (g) 9 •
Sat. Fat: (g) 3 • Cholesterol: (mg) 2 • Fiber: (g) 2 • Sodium: (mg) 139

Chocolate Marble Loaf

A great alternative to high fat and sugar-laden birthday cake recipes.

3 Tbl. cocoa
3 Tbl. soy — or rice milk
1 Tbl. molasses

---

2 1/2 cups spelt flour
1 1/4 cups Sucanat
1 1/2 tsp. baking powder
1 tsp. baking soda
1/4 tsp. salt

---

1 cup applesauce
1/3 cup plain yogurt
1/3 cup oil
2 tsp. vanila
2 egg whites
1 egg — or alternative

DIRECTIONS:

1. Mix cocoa, milk, molasses, and set aside.
2. Mix dry ingredients.
3. Mix liquids and stir into dry. Remove 1 cup batter, add to cocoa mixture and stir well.
4. Spoon cocoa batter alternately with vanilla into prepared 9" x 13" pan (or cupcake pans).
5. Bake at 350° for 35 to 45 minutes (about 20 – 25 minutes for cupcakes) or until done.

Makes 20 squares.

Calories: 142 • Protein: (g) 4 • Carbs: (g) 32 • Fat: (g) 1 •
Sat. Fat: (g) 0 • Cholesterol: (mg) 14 • Fiber: (g) 4 • Sodium: (mg) 93

Notes:

Not-to-be-Forgotten Extras

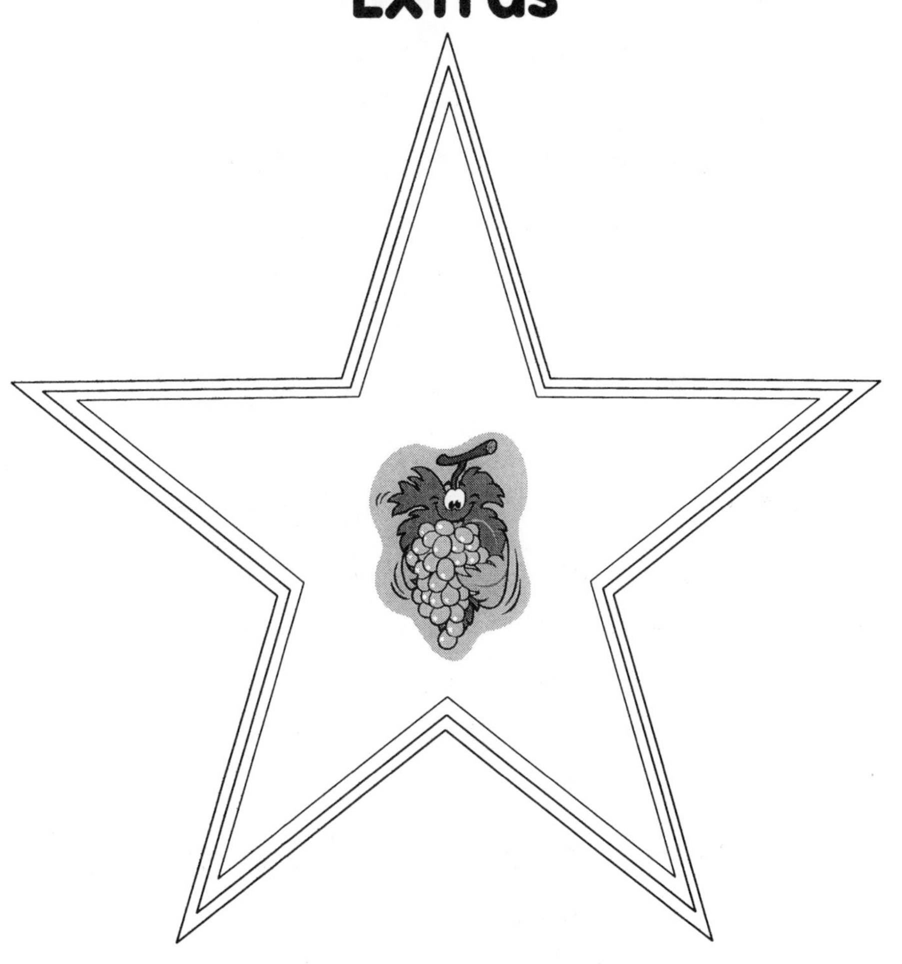

Power Pops
Banana Dogs
Fruit Kabobs
Banana Boats
Quick Grapes
Quick Sorbet
Trail Mix
Roasted Pumpkin Seeds
Baked Tortilla Chips
Nutty Dip
Onion Dip
Homemade Nut Butters
Pizza Mishaps
Power Packed Sandwich Spread
Dates & Nuts
Almond Crunch Bars
Haystacks
Almond Clusters
Space Balls
Honey Cinnamon Topping
Apple Syrup
Soda Substitute
Mineral Rich Fluid for Babies
Teething Cookies

Power Pops

8 oz. frozen fruit juice concentrate — or 2 cups fresh fruit
2 cups plain yogurt — or 2 pkg. Mori Nu Tofu, soft

DIRECTIONS:

1. Puree fresh fruit, if using.
2. Mix juice or fruit puree with yogurt or tofu. Pour into molds or small paper cups. If using cups, add craft sticks during freezing process for handles.

Makes approximately 9 pops.

Banana Dogs

An alternative to a PBJ sandwich with fruit. The bread and fruit are not the best food combination. This is a great idea for a picnic.

3/4 cup peanut butter — or almond butter
2 Tbl. honey — or maple syrup

---

4 spelt hot dog buns — or whole wheat

---

2 bananas
1 Tbl. lemon juice

DIRECTIONS:

1. Stir nut butter and honey together.
2. Place about 3 tablespoons of mixture on bun.
3. Peel the bananas. Cut in half lengthwise. Place on peanut butter mixture. Brush a little lemon juice over banana to keep it from browning.
4. Place top on sandwich. Wrap in plastic wrap.

Makes 4 sandwiches.

Fruit Kabobs

An easy version of a fruit salad that a child can make. A great idea for them to make for their own snack. Keep lots of fruit in the house so they have a big variety for their straws.

good variety of fruit

DIRECTIONS:

1. Wash fruit and cut into bite size pieces.
2. Push a straw through the pieces of fruit. If fruit is too hard, cut a hole with a knife.

NOTE:

☆ When a straw is pushed from the bottom through to the top of a strawberry, it automatically de-stems the strawberry.

Banana Boats

This quick easy recipe was donated by Jennifer Beck, children's nutritionist and author of the tape series, "Growing a Healthy Child."

1 peeled banana
toothpicks
1 bunch of grapes

---

1 long skewer
1 strawberry, halved

---

apple chunks

---

shredded coconut
blueberry juice

DIRECTIONS:

1. Stick toothpicks through peeled banana. Put grapes on the end to act as oars.
2. Insert skewer in the middle of the boat, straight up, to act as a mast.
3. Place strawberry on skewer to act as sail.
4. In the middle of the banana, put two toothpicks. Attach apple chunks to act as captain and shipmate.
5. Mix coconut with enough blueberry juice to color coconut blue. Put "dyed" coconut on plate. Put "boat" on the ocean of blue coconut.

Quick Grapes

An easy snack.

large bunch of seedless grapes

DIRECTIONS:

1. Remove grapes from stem. Place in storage bag and freeze.
2. Children can eat these frozen grapes like individual popsicles.
3. Do not give to toddler who can't chew or would swallow the grape whole.

Quick Sorbet

This dish is easy, delicious, and good for you!

various fruits (i.e., bananas, berries, grapes, pears, oranges, etc.), peeled, frozen

DIRECTIONS:

Mix frozen fruits in a blender or food processor for instant sorbet.

NOTE:

Variation:

☆ In a Champion juicer, frozen fruit can be used to make homogenized sorbet (all mixed together and quite smooth).

Trail Mix

Most children love trail mix. Let your children make their own.

various dried fruits (i.e., currants, raisins, figs, dates, pineapple chunks, banana chips, dates, etc.)
seeds (i.e., pumpkins, sesame, sunflower, etc.)
nuts (i.e., walnuts, almonds, cashews, chestnuts, etc.)

DIRECTIONS:

Mix all ingredients together.

NOTES:

☆ Trail mix can be added to yogurt, popsicles, or drizzled with the chocolate syrup recipe found in this book.

☆ If you buy trail mix, be sure to watch that the brand you select does not use hydrogenated fats/oils or that the dried fruits have used sulfites.

Roasted Pumpkin Seeds

A great way to use all of those pumpkin and/or squash seeds. A great family activity that produces a tasty, inexpensive, nutritional snack food.

1 cup seeds from freshly cut pumpkin or squash
1 tsp. olive oil — or canola oil
seasonings, as desired

DIRECTIONS:

1. Wash seeds and dry thoroughly.
2. Toss the seeds with oil (and any desired seasoning) and spread on a baking sheet.
3. Bake at 325° until desired crispness is reached. Stir occasionally.
4. Cool and store in refrigerator.

Makes 1 cup.

Baked Tortilla Chips

A quick, inexpensive alternative to fried chips.

1 pkg. plain tortillas (corn, whole wheat, or spelt)

---

sea salt — or salt-free seasoning
cayenne pepper — optional

DIRECTIONS:

1. Cut tortillas into quarters (or smaller wedges, if you are using large tortillas).
2. Place on ungreased cookie sheet in single layer. Bake at 350° for 4 minutes on each side or until crisp. (May take longer if tortilla is extra thick.)
3. Sprinkle with sea salt, cayenne, or any other herb mixture. Cool.

Makes 48 – 96 chips.

Nutty Dip

A great dip for veggies or fruit.

8 oz. Mori Nu Tofu, soft
4 Tbl. almond butter
2 Tbl. lemon juice — or to taste
1 1/2 Tbl. honey — or granulated sweetener

DIRECTIONS:

1. Blend all ingredients together in food processor.
2. Let chill, if time permits, to blend flavors.
3. Best if served at room temperature.

Makes 1 1/2 cups.

Onion Dip

A great dip for raw veggies or chips.

1/2 pkg. Mori Nu Tofu, soft
1 1/2 tsp. oil
1 Tbl. lemon juice
1 1/2 tsp. tahini — or milk
1 tsp. rice vinegar — or other vinegar
1/2 tsp. Umeboshi plum vinegar — or other vinegar
pinch of salt

----

1 small garlic clove
1/2 cup green onions, minced
1/2 cup mayonnaise
1/2 tsp. Worcestershire Sauce

DIRECTIONS:

1. Blend first 7 ingredients in blender until well blended.
2. Stir in garlic, onions, mayonnaise, and Worcestershire Sauce. Blend well and let chill for several hours, if time permits.

Makes 1 1/2 cups.

Homemade Nut Butters

Try the many easy varieties — even better than plain old peanut butter.

1 cup nuts (i.e., almonds, cashews, etc.) — or seeds

1/2 Tbl. flaxseed oil
1/2 Tbl. olive oil

---

1 – 2 Tbl. water, as needed

DIRECTIONS:

1. Grind nuts or seeds in high powered blender or food processor until powdered. A nut/seed grinder also works well.
2. Slowly add oil, with blender going until paste forms. If you have a good blender (i.e., a Bosch), you will need less oil and may need no additional oil.
3. Add water only to get desired consistency. Store in refrigerator.

Pizza Mishaps

This quick, easy recipe was donated by Jennifer Beck, children's nutritionist and author of the tape series, "Growing a Healthy Child."

1 toaster biscuit — or English muffin
spaghetti sauce

Toppings:
sliced olives, pineapple chunks, spinach, chopped tomatoes, chopped broccoli, sliced mushrooms, etc.

---

grated soy cheese — or raw milk cheese (Rella for soy or Alta Dena for raw milk)

DIRECTIONS:

1. Cover muffin or biscuit with sauce.
2. Cover with various toppings.
3. Sprinkle with cheese. Bake at 350° until cheese melts.

Power Packed Sandwich Spread

It's easy and good!

1/2 cup plain yogurt (soy or good dairy)
1/2 cup tahini (Arrowhead Mills or Maranatha)

DIRECTIONS:

1. Mix together.
2. Add any herbs to flavor, as desired.
3. Store in refrigerator.

Dates and Nuts

Try these for a delectable cookie.

1 cup pitted dates
1/4 cup currants — or raisins
1 cup pecans — or mixed, raw nuts
shredded coconut, optional
powdered soy — or tofu milk

DIRECTIONS:

1. Place into food processor. Mix until well blended.
2. Form into small balls. Roll in shredded coconut or powder.

Makes about 2 dozen cookies.

Almond Crunch Bars

A great variation on the old time Rice Krispy Treats. My family thinks these taste better!

1/2 cup brown rice syrup
1/2 cup almond butter
1/4 cup peanut butter
1 tsp. vanilla

1/2 cup chocolate chips without sugar
1/2 cup slivered almonds
1/2 cup Perky's Nutty Rice cereal
3 cups Barbara's Crispy Brown Rice cereal

DIRECTIONS:

1. Combine syrup and butters. Heat, on low, until mixture pulls away from the sides of the pan. Stir in vanilla.
2. Combine dry ingredients and add the syrup mixture. Spread into an oiled 9" x 13" pan. Pack down firmly. Let cool for a few minutes, then cut into squares. Refrigerate to set (cutting after totally hard is difficult).

Makes about 2 – 3 dozen bars.

Haystacks

An easy, unbaked cookie that can use carob or chocolate (sweetened or unsweetened chips). Kids love this and they can help make them.

1 pound carob chips — or chocolate chips (approx. 5 1/2 cups)

1/2 pound sunflower seeds (approximately 1 3/4 cups)
1/2 pound currants (approximately 2 cups)
1/4 pound slivered almonds (approximately 1 cup)

DIRECTIONS:

1. Melt chips.
2. Mix dry ingredients together. Stir in melted chip mixture and mix well.
3. Make little "haystacks" on oiled cookie sheet or cookie sheet lined with wax paper. Chill until set. Store in refrigerator.

Almond Clusters

A real favorite in my kid's cooking classes.

3 cups Oatio-type cereal
1 cup slivered almonds, ground
1/2 cup brown rice syrup
3 Tbl. almond butter — or cashew butter
1/2 tsp. vanilla
1/2 tsp. cinnamon

DIRECTIONS:

1. Mix all ingredients but cereal.
2. Stir in cereal and mix well.
3. Form into clusters and drop onto wax paper lined cookie sheet.
4. Chill.

NOTES:

Substitutions:

☆ Other cereals and nut butters can be used.

☆ Other spices can be used.

Makes about 3 – 4 dozen.

Space Balls

Even dedicated junk food junkies appreciate these.

2 cups almond butter
3/4 cup brown rice syrup
3/4 cup honey

---

1 cup oats
1 cup non-instant dry milk

---

4 – 7 cups mixed cereal

DIRECTIONS:

1. Soften almond butter and sweeteners. Mix together.
2. Blend oats in blender until smooth. Add milk to almond mixture. After well blended, add oat "flour."
3. Stir in enough cereal to make desired consistency. Form into balls and chill. Store in refrigerator.

NOTES:

☆ The cereal combination we like is: 2 – 4 cups Oatios, 2 cups Barbara's Brown Rice cereal, and 1 – 2 cups Perky's Nutty Rice cereal. The more cereal, the crunchier the cookie.

Substitution:

☆ Non-instant milk can be replaced with powdered soy or tofu milk.

Honey Cinnamon Topping

A great topping for pancakes and waffles that is different from the normal maple syrup, applesauce, or jam.

1 pkg. Mori Nu Tofu, soft drained
3 Tbl. honey
1/8 – 1/4 tsp. cinnamon

DIRECTIONS:

Blend all ingredients in blender until smooth.

Makes 1 cup.

Apple Syrup

An appetizing alternative to sugary syrups.

2 Tbl. arrowroot powder
1/2 tsp. cinnamon, ground

---

2 cups apple juice, unsweetened, unfiltered

DIRECTIONS:

1. Mix arrowroot and cinnamon.
2. Slowly pour in juice and mix well. Heat until thickened.
3. Serve over pancake wedges or squares.

Soda Substitute

This drink eliminates many of the harmful ingredients found in most sodas. It is also much less expensive.

quality juice
carbonated mineral water

DIRECTIONS:

1. Mix your child's favorite quality juice (even better with freshly squeezed juice) with carbonated mineral water.

NOTE:

☆ Adding 100 – 200 mg. of crushed vitamin C to this drink adds extra nutrition.

Mineral Rich Fluid for Babies

This fluid is rich in iron and various minerals.

1/4 cup organically grown almonds with skins
2 Tbl. organically grown oats
2 Tbl. organically grown raisins with no sulfites

DIRECTIONS:

1. Place in pint jar and cover with purified or distilled water.
2. Soak for two days in the refrigerator.
3. Strain liquid and store in refrigerator.
4. Serve warmed or cool.

Teething Cookies

A healthful alternative to most teething biscuits.

2 Tbl. brown rice syrup
2 Tbl. olive oil
1 Tbl. blackstrap molasses
1 egg yolk, beaten — or alternative

1/2 cup soy flour
1/4 cup fresh wheat germ
1/2 cup whole wheat flour — or alternative

DIRECTIONS:

1. Mix all liquid ingredients.
2. Mix all dry ingredients and then add to the liquid.
3. If too thick, add some soy milk to thin. If too thick, add more flour to stiffen.
4. Roll out 1/4" thick. Cut into rectangles. Place on cookie sheet. Bake at 350° for 15 – 20 minutes.

Makes about 48 cookies.

Part Four:

Resources

APPENDIX A

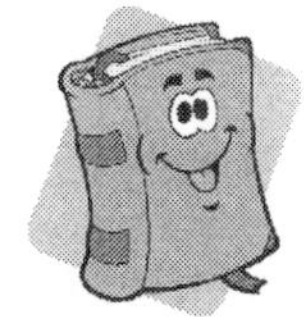

Resources for Children

After the Stork offers a wide variety of children's clothing made from natural fibers.

After the Stork
1501 12th Street NW
Albuquerque, NM 87104
(800) 333-5437

Autumn Harp offers talc-free baby powder, petroleum-free jelly, petroleum-free baby oil, and baby shampoo made from plant oils and herbs.

Autumn Harp
28 Rockydale Road.
Bristor, VT 05443
(802) 453-4807

Awareness Enterprises offers an audio cassette training series, "Growing a Healthy Child," by Jennifer Beck. Containing two 90 minute tapes and a resource planner, it is designed to help parents understand the basics of health and nutrition.

Awareness Enterprises
P.O. Box 1477
Beaverton, OR 97075
(503) 306-0707

Baby Bunz and Company offers a wide range of natural diapering products, including Nikkys and Dovetails; 100% cotton clothing for infants, wooden baby rattles, and dolls made from all-natural materials; lambskin booties, lambskin blankets.

Baby Bunz and Company
P.O. Box 1717
Sebastopol, CA 95473
(707) 829-5347

Biobottoms offers diapers, diaper covers, diaper duck for soiled diapers, an "It's easy to diaper with cloth" starter kit, 100% cotton clothing and shoes.

Biobottoms
Box 6009, 3820 Bodega Avenue
Petaluma, CA 94953
(707) 778-7945

Cot'n Kidz offers natural fiber clothing with standardized sizing and accessories for infants to 10 years.

Cot'n Kidz
P.O. Box 62000159
Newton, MA 01262
(617) 964-2686

Country Comfort offers natural baby care products.

Country Comfort
28537 Nuevo Valley Drive
P.O. Box 3
Nuevo, CA 92367
(800) 462-6617

Earth's Best Baby Food offers a selection of organic baby foods and cereals.

Earth's Best Baby Food
P.O. Box 887
Middlebury, VT 05753
(800) 442-4221

Family Clubhouse offers natural shampoos to eliminate lice.

Family Clubhouse
6 Chiles Avenue
Asheville, NC 28803
(603) 675-2055

Healthy Baby Supply Company offers a free catalog of natural baby products or a complimentary brochure on *Alternatives to Earaches*. Call or write Karen Kostohris at this address or number.

Healthy Baby Supply Company
323 E. Morton Street Dept. L
St. Paul, MN 55107
(612) 225-8535

Motherwear offers 100% cotton clothing and baby products.

Motherwear
P.O. Box 114
Northampton, MA 01061
(413) 586-3488

National Association of Diaper Services helps find diaper services in specific geographical areas.

National Association of Diaper Services
2017 Walnut Street
Philadelphia, PA 19103
(800) 462-6237

Natural Baby Company offers diaper products, natural toys, and other baby products.

Natural Baby Company
RDI, Box 160
Titusville, NJ 08560
(800) 388-BABY

Natural Lifestyle Supplies offers natural diaper products, natural toys, baby care products, and natural gift sets.

Natural Lifestyle Supplies
16 Lookout Drive
Asheville, NC 28804
(800) 752-2775

Perlinger Naturals offers natural baby foods.

Perlinger Naturals
238 Petaluma Avenue
Sebastopol, CA 95472
(707) 829-8363

Seventh Generation offers baby care products, sheets and other bedding, and natural baby wipes.

Seventh Generation
49 Hercules Drive
Colcheter, VT 05446
(800) 456-1177

Simply Pure Food offers organic strained and diced baby foods and cereals.

Simply Pure Food
RFD #3, Box 99
Bangor, ME 04401
(800) 426-7873

ALTERNATIVE HEALTH CARE RESOURCES

American Association of Naturopathic Physicians

2366 Eastlake Avenue, E
Seattle, WA 98102
(206) 323-7610

American College of Nurse-Midwives

1000 Vermont Avenue, NW
Washington, DC 20005
(202) 728-9860

American Holistic Medical Association

4101 Lake Boone Trail, Ste. 201
Raleigh, NC 27607
(919) 787-5146

American Osteopathic Association

142 E. Ontario Street
Chicago, IL 60611
(312) 280-5800

Bulimia Anorexia Self-Help, Inc.

522 N. New Ballas Road
St. Louis, MO 63141
(314) 567-4080

Feingold Association of the U.S.

P.O. Box 6550
Alexandria, VA 22306
(703) 768-3287

Homeopathic Academy of Naturopathic Physicians

4072 9th Avenue, NE
Seattle, WA 98105
(206) 547-9665

International College of Applied Kinesiology

P.O. Box 905
Lawrence, KS 66044
(913) 0542-1801

John Bastyr College of Naturopathic Medicine

144 NW 54th Street
Seattle, WA 98105
(206) 523-9585

La Leche League International

9816 Minneapolis Avenue
P.O. Box 1209
Franklin Park, IL 60131
1 (800) LALECHE

APPENDIX B

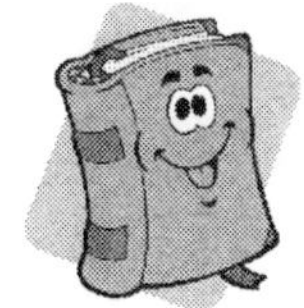

Supplementation for Kids

The following section is designed to help you know what products may be helpful in both the prevention and treatment of common childhood ailments. *The information provided is educational in nature, and is not intended to take the place of qualified diagnosis and treatment. Consult your chosen health professional for diagnosis, advice and treatment.*

DOSAGE

Two formulas for the calculation of herbal dosages for children are:

1. [Young's formula] Age in years ÷ (Age + 12) = portion of adult dose
2. Weight in pounds ÷ 150 = portion of adult dose

For example, if you have a 6 year old weighing 48 lb. who needs to take an herbal product where the adult dose is 15 drops taken 3 times a day you can calculate the child's dose in two different ways:

1. Young's formula
   (age in years) ÷ (6 (age) + 12) = 6/18 = 1/3 of adult dose
   1/3 of the adult dose would be 5 drops, 3 times a day
2. weight-based
   48 lb. ÷ 150 = 8/25 (.32 or a little less than 1/3)
   1/3 of the adult dose would be 5 drops, 3 times a day

(For math majors: the correct answer is 14.4 drops/day, the difference is not critical, but if it makes you feel better, you could leave out one drop.)

Why two formulas? For very young children (you might consult an expert anyway), weight is a better guide than age. Also, if a child is significantly off of the average weight curve, the weight-based formula is more accurate. By the way, adults who are larger or smaller than average should adjust their dosage as well, since the standard dose is based on the "average" 150 lb. male.

PREVENTATIVE STRATEGIES

Vitamins

If we were to give only one supplement to our daughter, it would be the *Mannatech* PhytoBears. These gummy bear shaped supplements contain Ambrotose™ (promotes cellular communication), flash-dried broccoli, brussels sprout, cabbage, carrot, cauliflower, garlic, kale, onion, papaya, pineapple, tomato and turnip in a base of gelatin and natural fruit fructose.

Research has shown these twelve fruits and vegetables to be some of the highest sources of phytochemicals, according to the American Cancer Society. Phytochemicals are plant chemicals that help build the immune system A strong immune system has the ability to keep cancer cells, as well as bacteria, fungus and infections in check.

Research has also linked these phytochemicals to marked reduction of ADHD symptoms (for a copy of the complete study, send a SASLE (self-addressed, stamped, legal envelope) to LFH.

PhytoBears can be purchased from LFH.

Protein Powders

If you want to add protein (vegetarian-based) to your diet, the following brands are excellent:

Nature's Life — Super-Green Pro-96

Naturade makes several protein powders, some with and some without soy

Nutribiotic Rice Protein (hypoallergenic)

These protein powders can be found in health food stores.

Greens Powders

Kyolic KyoGreen is a good blend of land and water based greens. These provide mild cleansing at the same time they supply easily assimilated nutrients. This is an excellent addition to a fruit smoothie.

KyoGreen can be found in local health food stores or ordered from LFH.

Friendly Bacteria (Acidophilus and Friends)

Lactobacillus acidophilus (and friends) are a group of friendly bacteria (probiotics) which colonize our digestive tracts. They actively fight against unhealthy bacteria, yeasts and molds which can cause digestive distress. Breast-fed infants get their first doses of probiotics from their mother's milk. Probiotics are especially important after a course of antibiotics, or if candida (thrush) is present.

LFH recommends Total Flora from *Infinity*. This is a capsule and can be taken by older children and adults.

Nature's Way Primadophilus comes in a powder form for young children ages 0 to 6 years (Primadophilus for Children), or a small size enteric coated capsule for older children 6 to 12 years old (Primadophilus Junior). Both products are dairy-free.

Nature's Life has a soy-based liquid acidophilus which comes in many flavors and is easy for younger children to take.

Natren also makes an excellent line of probiotics, including Life Start, which is specially formulated for infants.

Kyolic makes a product (KyoDophilus) that is especially useful for travel, since it does not require refrigeration to maintain potency. Because of the strains of acidophilus used, this product would be most appropriate for older children.

Cleansing

The subject of cleansing is covered in detail in my book *CLEANSING made simple*.

Mannatech makes MannaCleanse which is appropriate for teens and adults. For younger children PhytoBears by *Mannatech,* fresh juices and perhaps mild herbs under a health care provider's guidance can be helpful.

TREATMENT

Natural Antibiotic and Immune System Builders

Echinacea is an herb that stimulates the surface immune defenses. It is used to help fight infections, and to help reduce the number and severity of illnesses. It can be used for several months, if you take a week off every month. It should be used in combination with Astragalus for long-term immune building.

Gaia Herbs Echinacea glycerite (the strongest nonalcoholic echinacea I've found, but there is no flavoring)

HerbPharm Children's Echinacea (next strongest, and orange flavored — has weight-based dosage schedule on label)

Herbs for Kids Sweet Echinacea (generally well received by children — has age-based dosage schedule on label). Echinacea /Astragalus Blend is for long-term tonic use.

Echinacea/Goldenseal combinations are for shorter term use. Goldenseal is an herbal antibiotic (strong enough that you may need to take acidophilus afterward). It has toning properties for mucous membranes, making it a good bet with colds and sinus infections. It is probably not a good idea for infants (although I know mothers who have used it with good results). It definitely should not be used during pregnancy.

In short, the following brands are excellent:

Gaia Herbs Echinacea/Goldenseal glycerite

HerbPharm Golden Echinacea glycerite

Herbs for Kids Echinacea/Goldenseal Blend (flavored — has age-based dosage schedule on label)

Eclectic Institute Echinacea/Goldenseal glycerite (flavored)

Garlic is another herb that is good for the immune system, and can be taken all the time. Tests have shown that garlic has antibiotic properties. *Kyolic* makes an aged garlic product that is good for children — it is in liquid form. Older children could, of course, swallow the capsule form.

Flu and Fevers

For flu, fevers — *Herbs for Kids* Peppermint/Elder/Yarrow Blend is a variation on a traditional formula especially good during the early phases of a cold or flu. You can make a tea version of this at home.

Flu (and cold) Tea

peppermint leaves
elder blossoms
yarrow flowers
mullein leaves (for congestion) — optional

Mix equal parts of the above herbs together, and use 1 tsp. of the herb mixture for each cup of tea. The normal adult dosage would be 5 – 7 cups of tea a day. A 10 – 12 year old child could take 3 cups a day. Smaller children would take less than a cup of tea at a time — for example, a four year old child would get about 1 1/2 cups, broken up into 3 oz. servings taken 4 times a day.

Cough

Han's Natural Honey Loquat Syrup or *Boericke & Tafel* (B&T) Children's Cough & Bronchial Syrup (homeopathic) are useful for coughs.

Zand lozenges can also be used.

A homemade cough syrup can be just as effective, and fun to make as well.

Homemade Cough Syrup

1 tsp. lungwort
1 tsp. mullein
1 tsp. prickly ash bark
2 tsp. wild cherry bark

Pour 2 cups of boiling water over the herbs and let the mixture steep until cool. Strain and take 1 Tbl. every two hours, as needed (reduce this dosage for age or weight). Store the extra in refrigerator. Make a new batch of homemade cough syrup every two days.

Hayfever and Allergies

Eclectic Institute freeze-dried Nettles can be quite helpful — open the capsule for smaller children. *Herbs for Kids* Echinacea/Eyebright Blend is also good.

Quercetin, one of the bioflavonoids, can be helpful with hayfever and allergies as well.

Hidden food allergies might also be a problem.

Stomach Problems

For general problems, *Herbs for Kids* Minty Ginger Blend or *HerbPharm's* Children's Compound can be useful.

For motion sickness, ginger is very good (it tests better than those OTC pills). *New Moon Extracts* makes an organic ginger product in capsule, liquid extract, and syrup form.

Calming

Herbs for Kids makes Auntie Cham (a Chamomile-based formula) and Uncle Val (with Valerian). These can be used for occasional sleeplessness or tension.

Planetary Formulas makes Calm Child, which some parents have found to be helpful.

Bach Rescue Remedy is very good for stressful situations.

Dietary changes (for possible food allergies) can really make a difference.

REMEDIES FOR EXTERNAL USE

For general healing and dry skin *Mannatech* Emprizone with aloe vera can be helpful.

Drawing salve (black salve/ointment) can be used for splinters, boils, and swollen glands. *Nature's Way* Black Ointment or Icthammol Ointment are two possibilities.

For diaper rash try *Weleda* Diaper-Care (a zinc & calendula baby ointment).

Eyes

For pink eye, *HerbPharm* makes an herbal eyewash. You will need to dilute it with saline solution (directions on the bottle) and use it in an eye cup.

For dry or allergic eyes *Similasan* makes two homeopathic eye drops.

Skin

For psoriasis or eczema try *Enzymatic Therapy's* Simicort (external application). This product may be too strong for small children. These skin conditions may be caused by a deficiency of essential fatty acids — good sources of essential fatty acids include flaxseed oil or evening primrose oil. Vitamin E may also be helpful. Another common cause of skin problems is food allergies.

Cold Sores/Fever Blisters/Canker Sores

Enzymatic Therapy's Herpilyn is good for external application to cold sores or fever blisters. Dietary changes may also be helpful. Chocolate, nuts, and some other foods have a high ratio of the amino acid arginine to lysine — this can encourage growth of the virus that causes cold sores.

I put canker sores in this section even though they are very different — these are the little white ulcers inside the mouth, and they hurt. There is a good chance that food allergies play a part in canker sores. DGL licorice can help with them — it is good for ulcers anywhere in the digestive tract. Acidophilus can also be helpful.

Itching/Chicken Pox

Some people have found relief using *Enzymatic Therapy* Herpilyn on chicken pox, but that can be expensive if a large portion of the body is involved.

Here is a bath recipe that will help with itching or dry, irritated skin:

Oatmeal and Herb Bath Bag

7/8 cup rolled oats
2 Tbl. blanched almonds
2 Tbl. chickweed
2 Tbl. nettles

2 Tbl. plantain
2 Tbl. calendula

Whirl rolled oats and blanched almonds together in a blender. Combine the resulting mixture with chickweed, nettles, plantain, and calendula (the herbs are optional, but have all been traditionally known to reduce itching or heal skin). Put the mixture in a double layer of cheesecloth and tie securely. Allow the water to run over the bag, or pour boiling water over the bag and then fill the tub.

Acne

Teens often have skin problems due, in part, to hormonal changes. Actually, poor food choices and stored toxins have been building in the lymph and the liver. These, added to the hormonal stress, combine for a double whammy. If you have already been making the appropriate dietary changes, now would be a good time to start skin brushing for lymph cleansing (this is too rough for younger skin). Use a natural bristle brush (available at health food stores). Start brushing in small circles from the extremities in toward your heart. Follow the brushing with a shower to remove the loosened, dead skin cells. Good herbs to try would be dandelion and yellow dock (used as teas). *Gaia Herbs* makes Milk Thistle/Yellow Dock Supreme for this purpose. For external application, Emprizone from *Mannatech* can be excellent. It can be ordered from LFH.

Earache

Gaia Herbs Mullein/Hypericum Flower oil (which contains organic garlic) is among the strongest products. Parents have thanked me for recommending this. To use, slightly warm the oil and put two or three drops in the effected ear. If necessary, put a piece of a cotton ball in the ear to keep the warm oil from draining out. See chapter 9 for more details on earaches.

Teething

For teething problems the following products are excellent:

Herbs for Kids Gum-omile Oil — topical application
Hylands teething tablets (homeopathic)

ADDITIONAL HELPFUL HINTS

- ••• Herbs are best taken on an empty stomach.
- ••• Vitamins are best taken with meals and earlier in the day is better.
- ••• Minerals are best taken apart from whole grains, which can block absorption.
- ••• Minerals can be taken in the evening.
- ••• Iron taken with Vitamin C absorbs better.
- ••• Copper and zinc can block each other's absorption, but increased zinc intake will require copper supplementation, as well.
- ••• It is good to give rest time to your child's body, maybe a day or two off of herbs and supplements each week. Don't do this in the middle of an acute illness.
- ••• Liquid vitamins or herbs can be mixed with a small amount of water or juice, but it is not a good idea to put them in a baby's bottle.
- ••• Many parents are afraid their children won't get enough calcium (or protein, or iron…) if they switch to a total vegetarian diet. While it is possible to cause problems here, it is also possible to miss these nutrients (or at least their proper absorption) consuming a diet containing dairy and meat. Investigate food sources of nutrients — like kale for calcium or nuts and seeds (pistachio, pinon, sesame, sunflower, and pumpkin) for iron. In addition, good supplements for children are available.

PREFERRED SUPPLEMENT, HERB, & HOMEOPATHIC COMPANIES

Bach Flower Remedies
Oxfordshire OX14 5JX
England

Boericke & Tafel, Inc.
1011 Arch Street
Philadelphia, PA 19107
215-922-2967

Eclectic Institute, Inc.
14385 SE Lusted Road
Sandy, Oregon 97055
800-332-HERB

Enzymatic Therapy
825 Challenger Drive
Green Bay, WI 54311
800-783-2286

Gaia Herbs
12 Lancaster County Road
Harvard, MA 01451
800-831-7780

Han's is imported by:
Prince of Peace Ent., Inc.
3450 3rd St. Ste. #3G
San Francisco, CA 94124
800-732-2328

Herbs for Kids
151 Evergreen Drive, Ste. D
Bozeman, MT 59715
406-587-0180
fax: 406-587-0111

HerbPharm

PO Box 116
Williams, OR 97544
800-348-HERB

Hylands (Standard Homeopathic Company)

PO Box 61604
Los Angeles, CA 90014
213-321-4284

(Kyolic) Wakunaga of America Co., Ltd.

23501 Madero
Mission Viejo, CA 92691
714-855-2776

Mannatech is available from:

Lifestyle for Health

8122 SouthPark Lane
Littleton, CO 80120
303-794-4477
fax: 303-794-1449

McZand Herbal, Inc.

PO Box 5312
Santa Monica, CA 90409
310-822-0500

Natren, Inc.

3105 Willow Lane
Westlake Village, CA 91361
805-371-4742

Naturade Product's, Inc.

Paramount, CA 90723

Nature's Life

Garden Grove, CA 90630
800-854-6837

Nature's Way Products, Inc.

10 Mountain Springs Parkway
PO Box 4000
Springville, Utah 84663
800-9-NATURE

New Chapter, Inc./New Moon Extracts

99 Main Street
Brattleboro, VT 05301
800-543-7279

Nutribiotic

PO Box 238
Lakeport, CA 95453
707-263-0411
PO Box 600
800-635-1233

Raw Materials Food Company

PO Box 18932
Boulder, CO 80308-1932
303-499-7403

Similasan Corp.

Kent, WA 98032
800-426-1644

Weleda, Inc.

PO Box 249
Congers, NY 10920

NOTE

While all of these products are good quality, we do not necessarily endorse the philosophy or spirituality of these companies. The recommendations here are based on training and product experience. This is not a comprehensive list, there are many good products not listed here.

The information in this appendix has been compiled by Ed Hinckley and Cheryl Townsley.

APPENDIX C

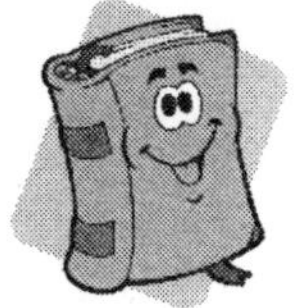

Preferred Brands

When a person begins to change what he or she eats, one of the most overwhelming jobs is going grocery shopping. The more familiar brands go by the wayside. But how does one even begin to shop for new brands? Our family has found the following brands taste good, are reasonably priced, and contain quality ingredients. It is important to support companies that are committed to quality products — to do our part to make sure they're healthy, also.

This list is not all-inclusive, but it does contain the food brands we use on a regular basis. I am sure you will find these brands to be a good starting place for your nutritional journey. No company has paid for these recommendations. Rather, I am simply passing on our preferences after many years of continuous experimentation.

If you are unable to find these products in your store, you may want to ask that they carry them. Some companies allow you to order their pproducts directly. Many have free recipe booklets and product brochures.

Alta Dena has a great line of quality dairy products, from fresh milk to kefir, yogurt, ice cream and others. They are committed to producing milk products without using bovine growth hormones. Dairy products without this hormone are safer for you and your family. Alta Dena's quality and integrity are excellent.

Alta Dena Certified Dairy
17637 Valley Boulevard
City Industry, CA 91744-5731
phone: 818-964-6401
fax: 818-965-1960

Annie's produces excellent dressings and barbecue sauces. Their dressings and sauces are just like homemade — fresh and tasty. Try their barbecue sauce on oven-fried potatoes. The raspberry dressing is one of our family's favorites.

Annie's
Foster Hill Road
North Calais, VT 05650
phone: 802-456-8866

Arrowhead Mills is a wonderful manufacturer that will easily replace many all-purpose brands that you currently purchase. Virtually all their products are organic with great taste and include whole grains, flours, mixes, beans, seeds, nut and seed butters (they have excellent tahini), oils, flakes and soup mixes.

Arrowhead Mills, Inc.
110 South Lawton
Box 2059
Hereford, TX 79045
phone: 806-364-0730

Barbara's Bakery provides quality, nutritious foods, from chips, pretzels and cookies to cereals, granola bars, bread sticks and crackers. Their food is tasty and very reasonably priced. Many low-fat and no-fat foods are available.

Barbara's Bakery, Inc.
3900 Cypress Drive
Petaluma, CA 94954
phone: 707-765-2273

Barlean's is my very favorite source of flaxseed oil. Their integrity and their commitment to organic, quality products make them a leader in the industry. Their products are available in the more well known oil form or in a capsule form. Store all of their products in the refrigerator and use them before the expiration date.

Barlean's
4936 Lake Terrell Road
Ferndale, WA 98248
phone: 619-484-1035

Cascadian Farm provides a wealth of excellent products. Many of their products are organic, from their frozen fruits and vegetables to their jams, jellies, preserves, sorbets, pickles and relishes. They have great "popsicles" made with organic milk and unrefined sugar. They have Kosher foods.

Cascadian Farm
P.O. Box 568
Concrete, WA 98237
phone: 206-855-0100
fax: 206-855-0444

Celestial Seasonings produces the finest herbal teas. They now also have a line of black teas and gourmet after-dinner teas. Any of their teas mix well with fresh fruit juices for another delightful option.

Celestial Seasonings
4600 Sleepytime Drive
Boulder, CO 80020
phone: 303-530-5300

Cold Mountain Miso (white miso) can be found in the dairy sections of most health food stores. The lighter the color of the miso, the milder the flavor. Miso is a great replacement for traditional bouillon cubes.

Cold Mountain Miso
Miyako Oriental Foods Inc.
4287 Puente Avenue
Baldwin Park, CA 91706
phone: 818-962-9633
fax: 818-814-4569

Coleman Natural Meats come from cattle raised without hormones or steroids. The flavor is beyond comparison with other commercially available meats. They have beef and other meats.

Coleman Natural Meats Inc.
5140 Race Court #4
Denver, CO 80127
phone: 303-297-9393
fax: 303-297-0426

DeBoles Pasta is a good transition pasta for families just beginning to change their diets. These pastas are made with semolina and Jerusalem artichoke flours. They have some corn pasta and other bakery products. This pasta is much lighter than white flour pasta. It comes in many varieties.

DeBoles Nutritional Foods, Inc.
2120 Jericho Turnpike
Garden City Park, NY 11040
phone: 516-742-1818

Enzymatic Therapy is a line of supplements found in health food stores. I recommend it as the first place to start when looking for a supplement in a store. They have supplements and homeopathics under the name of Lehning. They are committed to quality and integrity.

Enzymatic Therapy
825 Challenger Drive
Green Bay, WI 54311
phone: 800-783-2286
fax: 414-469-4400

French Meadow provides a full line of deliciously different breads made of alternative flours, many of which are also yeast-free. They may often be found in the freezer section of local health food stores. Their spelt, yeast-free pizza crusts are quite tasty.

French Meadow
2610 Lyndale Avenue South
Minneapolis, MN 55408
phone: 612-870-4740

Frontier provides fresh herbs in both bulk and packaged forms. They also produce organic coffees. This company is committed to quality and integrity.

Frontier Cooperatives Herbs
1 Frontier Road
P.O. Box 299
Norway, IA 52318
phone: 800-669-3275

FruitSource is a balanced sweetener made from brown rice and grapes that some diabetics can use. It comes in both liquid and granular forms. It can be used in a one for one ratio for sugar replacement. Due to its humectancy, fat in recipes using FruitSource should be reduced. Check the FruitSource label for guidelines.

FruitSource
1803 Mission Street, #404
Santa Cruz, CA 95060
phone: 408-457-1136

Garden of Eatin' has a wide variety of chips. I have found that many people do better with the blue or red corn chips instead of the yellow. They also have excellent pita breads, bagels, tortillas, chapatis and sprouted rolls. Certified organic ingredients are included in most products.

Garden of Eatin'
5300 Santa Monica Boulevard
Los Angeles, CA 90029
phone: 213-462-5406

Horizon is a supplier of dairy products that are all organic. It is cow, and not goat, based. They carry a full line of milk, cheese and yogurt.

Horizon
Boulder, CO 80301

Imagine Foods makes three delicious brands, including Rice Dream, Ken & Robert's and Veggie Pockets. Rice Dream is a food product made from the starch portion of brown rice. It is a delicious milk that can be used for drinking, cooking and baking. It is also available in frozen "ice-cream" type products. Ken & Robert's is a brand of delicious frozen vegetarian entrees. Veggie Pockets are frozen vegetarian pocket sandwiches, individually frozen for quick meals.

Imagine Foods
350 Cambridge Avenue, #350
Palo Alto, CA 94306
phone: 415-327-1444
fax: 415-327-1459

Knudsen & Sons supplies great juices, carbonated beverages, syrups and spreads. Their line of products are excellent replacements for less healthful sugar-sweetened colas and carbonated beverages.

Knudsen & Sons
P.O. Box 369
Chico, CA 95927
phone: 916-891-1517

Kyolic products are a daily staple in our home. From Kyolic (aged garlic) to KyoGreen powder, we use each product to build up our immune systems and maintain strong body systems. We add KyoGreen powder to our fruit smoothies each morning. Kyolic oderless aged garlic is a regular supplement all year long, especially during fall and winter. We use KyoDophilus (acidophilus) to balance intestinal flora (especially important after a round of antibiotics or having colonics).

Wakunaga of America Co., Ltd.
23501 Madero
Mission Viejo, CA 92691
phone: 714-855-2776

Lundberg produces organic and premium brown-rice products. They also have rice blends, brown-rice cakes, flours, cereals and pilafs. Their brown-rice syrup is an excellent sugar replacement that many diabetics can use. Their brown-rice pudding mixes are excellent, as are their one-step chili mixes.

Lundberg Family Farms
P.O. Box 369
Richvale, CA 95974
phone: 916-882-4551

Maine Coast Sea Vegetables offers a full line of sea vegetables or seaweed. Adding that strip of kombu to your soups or beans aids in digestion and intake of minerals.

Maine Coast Sea Vegetables
Shore Road
Franklin, MA 04630
phone: 207-565-2144

Mom's Spaghetti Sauce is one of our all-time favorite sauces to use on our homemade pasta. It is swimming with big chunks of fresh basil and whole cloves of garlic. This is a truly delicious sauce.

Mom's Spaghetti Sauce
Timpone's Fresh Foods Corp.
3708 Woodbury
Austin, TX 78704
phone: 512-442-7773

Mori Nu has the best silken tofu (a smooth tofu with the texture of sour cream, without the cholesterol). It works the best with many of my recipes. It comes in aseptic packaging for longer shelf life. Their "lite" tofu has the least amount of fat of any tofu on the market.

Mori Nu
2050 West 190th, #110
Torrance, CA 90504
phone: 800-NOW TOFU
fax: 310-787-2727

Mountain Sun is committed to organic products. They provide great organic and natural food juices under the labels of Mountain Sun and Apple Hill. Their flavors and varieties are superb.

Mountain Sun
18390 Highway 145
Dolores, CO 81323
phone: 303-882-2283
fax: 303-882-2270

Muir Glen tomato products are by far my favorite. These organically grown tomato products are packaged in enamel lined cans, which produces a superior taste and product. Their products range from chunky sauces to paste to whole tomatoes. Throw away those tinny-tasting tomatoes and try Muir Glen.

Muir Glen
424 North 7th Street
Sacramento, CA 95814
phone: 800-832-6345
fax: 916-557-0903

Nayonaise produces a dairy-free mayo made from tofu. They also make delicious tofu dressings, wonton skins, egg roll wrappers and tofu.

Nasoya Foods Inc.
23 Jytek Drive
Leominster, MA 01453
phone: 508-537-0713

Nest Eggs provides eggs from uncaged hens that are fed a drug-free diet. Quality eggs are just as important as organic grains, produce and meats.

Nest Eggs Inc.
P.O. Box 14599
Chicago, IL 60614

Pamela's Products produces our favorite cookies. Many of their cookies are wheat-free (wheat is the most common American food allergy), sugar-free and some are dairy-free. A line of biscotti cookies has been added to the regular line.

Pamela's Products
156 Utah Avenue
South San Francisco, CA 94080
phone: 415-952-4546

Redwood provides a tasty goat yogurt product. Goat yogurt is much easier for me to digest than cow's yogurt.

Redwood
10855 Occidental Road
Sebastopol, CA 95472
phone: 707-823-8250

Roaster Fresh makes an excellent line of nut butters. They are produced by Kettel Foods, which also makes chips, popcorn and other nuts and seeds.

Roaster Fresh/Kettle Foods
P.O. Box 664
Salem, OR 97308
phone: 503-364-0399

San-J has great sauces for stir-fries and marinades. Their tamari has an excellent flavor and will quickly replace your sodium-laden soy sauces. Their Thai peanut sauce is great for stir-fries and in salads. Their miso soup (I prefer the mild) is a delicious cup-a-soup.

San-J International, Inc.
2880 Sprouse Drive
Richmond, VA 23231
phone: 804-226-8333

Sharon's Finest produces Rella, a line of soy cheeses for those with dairy sensitivities. All Rella cheeses work great as alternatives to dairy-based cheese. Rella melts well and has good flavor. They have many varieties in their line.

Sharon's Finest
P.O. Box 5020
Santa Rosa, CA 95402
phone: 707-576-7050

Shelton poultry products are free-range grown, raised without antibiotics, hormones, or growth stimulants — which are common in most other commercially raised chickens and turkeys. ("All Natural" on a poultry label is defined by the Department of Agriculture as "minimally processed with no artificial ingredients." This claim on a whole bird only means that the bird has not been artificially basted, which is basically meaningless.) Shelton provides fresh poultry and other poultry-related products. Their chicken broth is excellent.

Shelton Poultry
204 Loranne
Pomona, CA 91767
phone: 909-623-4361

Sno-Pac provides a line of reasonably priced, organic frozen vegetables. Out with the old brands, loaded with chemicals, and in with Sno-Pac.

Sno-Pac Foods Inc.
379 S. Pine Street
Caledonia, MN 55921
phone: 507-724-5285

Spectrum Naturals' oils are expeller pressed without solvents. Both refined and unrefined oils are available. Their products range from oils and supplemental oils to cheese, mayonnaise, vinegars, dressings and sauces. Their brand names include Spectrum Naturals (oils), Veg-Omega, Sonnet Farms (cheese), Ayla's Organic (dressings) and Blue Banner.

Spectrum Naturals, Inc.
133 Copeland Street
Petaluma, CA 94952
phone: 707-778-8900
fax: 707-765-1026

Sucanat is a sweetener using dehydrated cane juice. All of the minerals contained in molasses are found in Sucanat. It can be found in regular and a honey version which is a little lighter in color and flavor. It is a favorite for cooking and for sweetening beverages.

Sucanat
P.O. Box 2860
Dayton Beach, FL 32120
phone: 904-258-4707

Sunspire is your answer to sugar-laden chocolate. Sunspire products contain no refined sugar and have a great taste. They can be purchased in carob, chocolate, mint and peanut. They provide confections and chocolate chips. They also have many dairy-free products.

Sunspire
2114 Adams Avenue
San Leandro, CA 94577
phone: 510-569-9731

Trace Minerals provides several mineral products that we find to be excellent. We recommend their ConcenTrace Mineral Drops and their Arth-X product (for help with arthritis pain and symptoms).

Trace Minerals
1990 West 330 South
Ogden, UT 84401
phone: 800-624-7145

VitaSpelt produces some of the best whole-grain pastas. They use whole-grain spelt, which many wheat-sensitive people can tolerate. Be sure to not overcook whole-grain pasta, as that will make it mushy. They have added a new focacia bread, which can be used as an excellent pizza base. I have prepared many recipes for VitaSpelt products.

VitaSpelt
Purity Foods Inc.
2871 West Jolly Road
Okemos, MI 48864
phone: 800-99-SPELT

Westbrae and Little Bear are two excellent brands. The company is committed to organic and low-fat products. Little Bear, under the brand name Bearitos, has excellent chips, taco shells, tostada shells, popcorn, salsa, refried beans and pretzels. They also produce a licorice without refined sugar and additives. Westbrae has excellent snack food, cookies, soy milk, soy beverages and condiments.

Little Bear/Westbrae
1065 East Walnut Street
Carson, CA 90746
phone: 310-886-8219

APPENDIX D

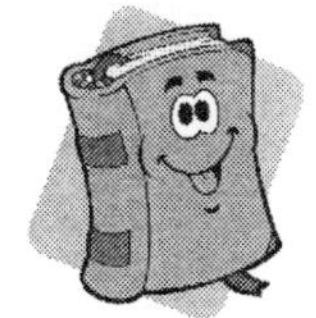

Substitutions and Equivalents

Fruit Equivalents:

Apples: 3 medium = 1 lb. = 3 c. sliced

Bananas: 3 medium = 1 lb. = 2 c. sliced = 1 c. mashed

Dates: 1 lb. = 3 c. chopped

Lemon: 1 medium = 2 to 3 Tbl. juice, 2 tsp. lemon zest

Lime: 1 medium = 1 1/2 to 2 Tbl. juice, 1 tsp. lime zest

Orange: 1 medium = 1 1/2 c. juice, 2 tsp. orange zest

Peach: 1 medium = 1 1/2 c. sliced

Pear: 1 medium = 1 1/2 c. sliced

Raisins: 1 lb. = 3 c.

Strawberries: 1 qt. = 4 c. sliced

Grain Equivalents:

Cornmeal: 1 lb. = 3 c.

Flaked cereal: 3 c. dry = 1 c. crushed

Oats: 1 c. = 1 3/4 c. cooked

Rice: 1 c. = 3 to 4 c. cooked

Nut Equivalents:

Almonds: 1 lb. unshelled = 1 3/4 c. nutmeat
1 lb. shelled = 3 1/2 c. nutmeat

Peanuts: 1 lb. unshelled = 1 3/4 c. nutmeat
1 lb. shelled = 3 1/2 c. nutmeat

Pecans: 1 lb. unshelled = 1 3/4 c. nutmeat
1 lb. shelled = 3 1/2 c. nutmeat

Walnuts: 1 lb. unshelled = 1 3/4 c. nutmeat
1 lb. shelled = 3 1/2 c. nutmeat

Vegetable Equivalents:

Cabbage: 1 lb. = 3 c. shredded

Corn: 2 medium ears = 1 c. kernels

Mushrooms: 8 oz. = 3 c. raw = 1 c. sliced, cooked

Onion: 1 medium = 1/2 c. chopped

Pepper, green: 1 large = 1 c. diced

Potato (sweet): 3 medium = 3 c. sliced

Potato (white): 3 medium = 2 c. cubed, cooked = 1 3/4 c. mashed

Other Equivalents:

Carob chips: 12 oz. = 2 c.

Carob powder: 1 lb. = 4 c.

Coconut: 1 lb. = 5 c. flaked or shredded

Milk cheese, raw: 1 lb. = 4 c. shredded

Pasta: 4 oz. = 1 c. = 2 1/4 c. cooked

General Equivalents:

3 tsp. = 1 Tbl.

16 fluid oz. = 2 c. = 1 pt.

2 Tbl. (liquid) = 1 oz.

1/8 c. = 2 Tbl.

4 Tbl. = 1/4 c.

5 1/3 Tbl. = 1/3 c.

8 Tbl. = 1/2 c.

16 Tbl. = 1 c.

8 fluid oz. = 1 c.

1/3 c. = 5 Tbl. + 1 tsp.

2/3 c. = 10 Tbl. + 2 tsp.

4 c. = 1 qt.

4 qts. = 1 gal.

Substitutes:

Baking powder: two parts cream of tartar, one part baking soda, and two parts arrowroot

Bread crumbs: toasted oats, sesame seeds, cooked brown rice, or other cracked grains

Butter: in baking, canola oil, safflower oil, sunflower oil, or applesauce (up to 1/2 c. per recipe)

1 Tbl. = 1 tsp. light miso plus 2 tsp. olive oil for mashed potatoes

Buttermilk: 1 c. = 1 c. minus 1 Tbl. of soy milk, rice milk, or almond milk, plus 1 Tbl. lemon juice

Cheese: equal amounts of soy or almond cheeses.

Cheese, cottage cheese:

1 lb. firm tofu, mashed
1 Tbl. olive oil
1 Tbl. rice or apple-cider vinegar
2 Tbl. lemon juice
1/4 to 1/2 tsp. onion powder, to taste
1/4 to 1/2 tsp. salt or tamari, to taste

Mix half of tofu and remaining ingredients in blender. Mix in remaining mashed tofu.

Cheese, cream cheese = "yo" cheese: Strain yogurt in yogurt strainer, or coffee filter placed in strainer, for 24 hours (set in refrigerator while draining).

Cheese, ricotta:

1 lb. firm tofu, mashed
1/4 c. olive oil
1/2 tsp. nutmeg
1/2 tsp. salt or tamari

Mix half of tofu and remaining ingredients in blender. Mix in remaining tofu.

Chicken: (This tip was provided us by Morinaga, manufacturers of Mori Nu Tofu.) Slice one package of Mori Nu Extra Firm Tofu, "lite" into four horizontal slices. Freeze in a single layer. Thaw and squeeze out excess liquid. Marinate in a sauce for 30 minutes or more. Cook according to the individual recipe's directions.

Chocolate: 1 square or 1 oz. = 3 Tbl. carob plus 1 Tbl. oil and 1 Tbl. water

Cocoa: 1 c. = 1 c. carob powder
Cornstarch: 1 Tbl. = 1 Tbl. arrowroot powder

Cream, heavy: 1 Tbl. tahini dissolved in 1/4 c. water (this will not whip)

Cream, sour: "yo" cheese or equal amount of soft tofu

Currants: raisins

Eggs: one egg =

1 Tbl. soy flour
1 Tbl. water plus 1 Tbl. powdered soy lecithin
commercial egg replacer
half of a ripe banana
4 oz. firm tofu
1/4 c. applesauce
1/4 c. "yo" cheese

Flour, white (as sauce thickener): 1 Tbl. = 1/2 Tbl. arrowroot

Flour, white (in baking):

1 c. = 1 c. corn flour
1 c. = 3/4 c. coarse cornmeal
1 c. = 7/8 c. rice flour
1 c. = 1 c. spelt flour
1 c. = 1 c. kamut flour
1 c. = 1/2 c. barley flour + 1/4 c. rice flour + 1/2 Tbl. arrowroot powder

Garlic: 1 clove =

1 tsp. minced garlic
1/2 tsp. garlic powder

Milk: 1 c. = 1 c. almond milk, soy milk, rice milk, or 1 c. water plus 1 Tbl. tahini, mixed

Milk, sour: 1 c. = 1 Tbl. lemon juice or vinegar plus 1 c. less 1 Tbl. milk. Let set 5 minutes.

Pan preparation: lightly oil or brush with lecithin mixture (6 Tbl. canola, 2 Tbl. liquid lecithin — mix well).

Pepper: 1 tsp. black pepper = 1/4 tsp. cayenne

Sugar, brown:

1 c. = 1/2 c. date sugar and 1/2 c. honey
1 c. = 1/2 to 3/4 c. honey
1 c. = 3/4 c. maple syrup

(use 1/2 c. less liquid per cup sweetener and reduce oven temperature by 25 degrees)

Sugar, white:

1 c. = 1 c. FruitSource
1 c. = 3/4 c. to 1 c. Sucanat
1 c. = 3/4 c. maple syrup (use 2 Tbl. less liquid in recipe)
1 c. = 3/4 c. honey (use 2 Tbl. less liquid per cup of honey used and lower oven temperature by 25 degrees)
1 c. = 1 c. rice syrup
1 c. = 1 c. molasses plus 1/2 tsp. baking soda (use 1/4 c. less recipe liquid per 1 c. of molasses)

Worcestershire sauce: 3 Tbl. = 1/4 c. tamari

Yogurt: equal amount of tofu

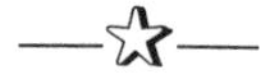

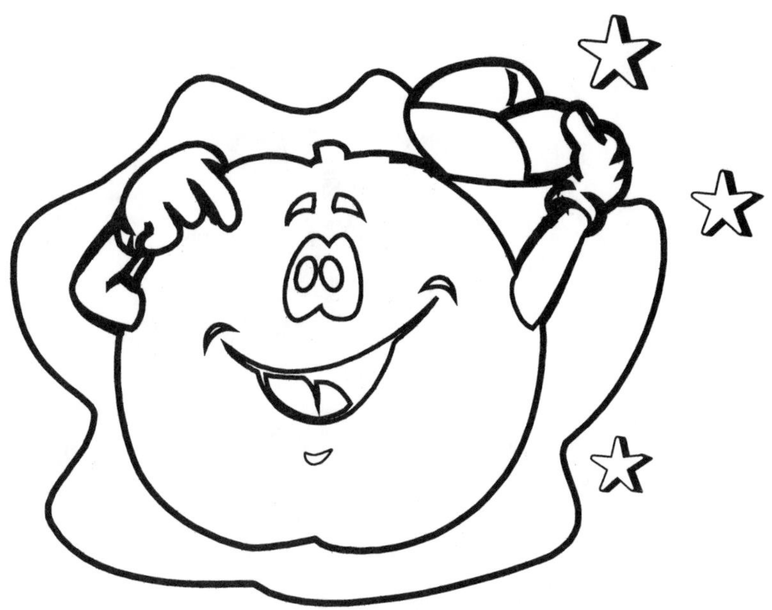

Hi! My name is Peter Peach. My friends and I would like to help you. Can you guess how?

Hi! I'm Sarah Strawberry. I don't like it when I get sick, do you? I can help you get strong and fight off yucky germs! With my help you can beat them cold.

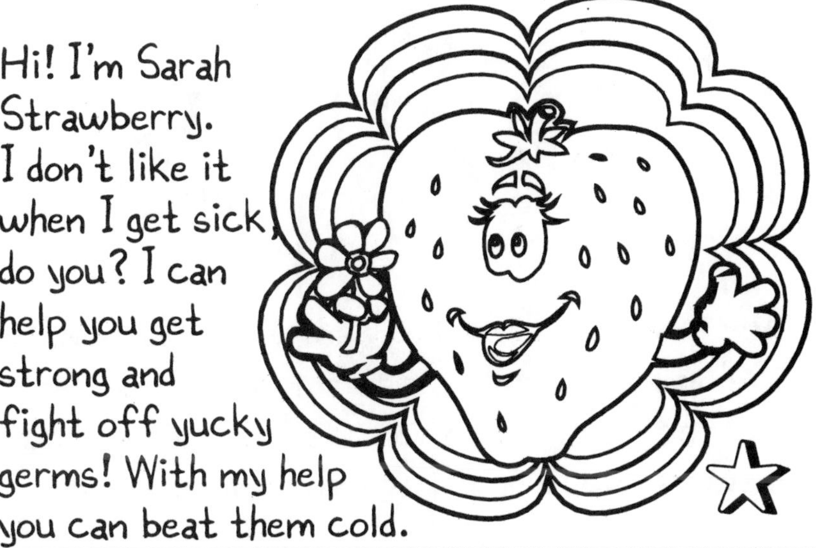

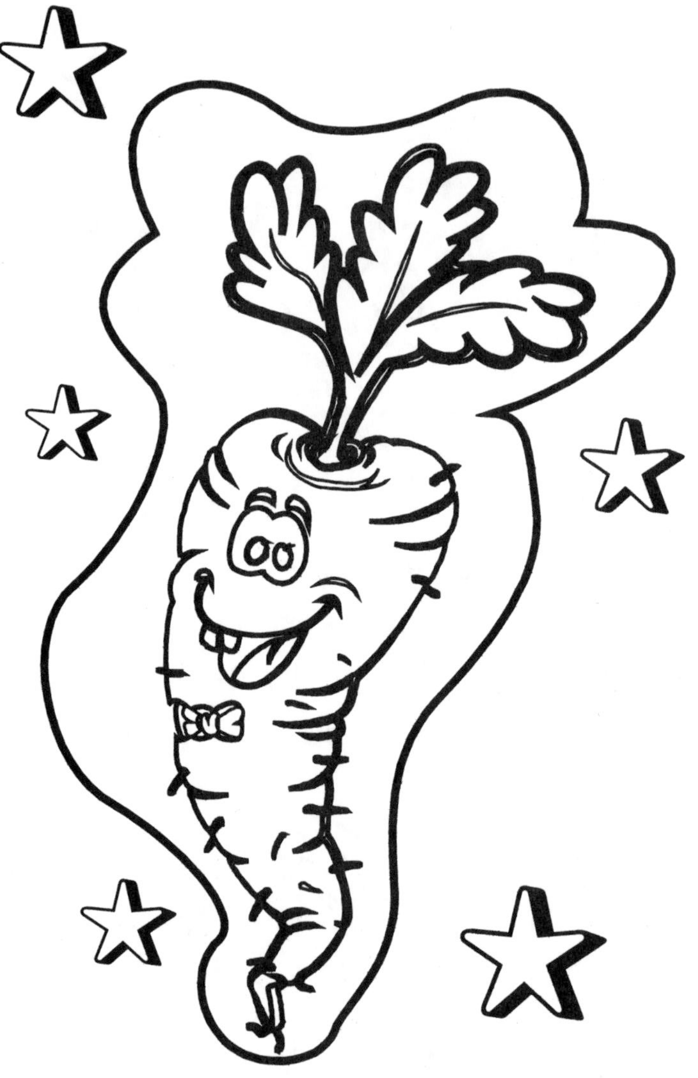

And I'm Carl Carrot. I can help you a bunch. Did you know that I can help your eyes see better – even when you are in the dark. You never know when that will come in handy!

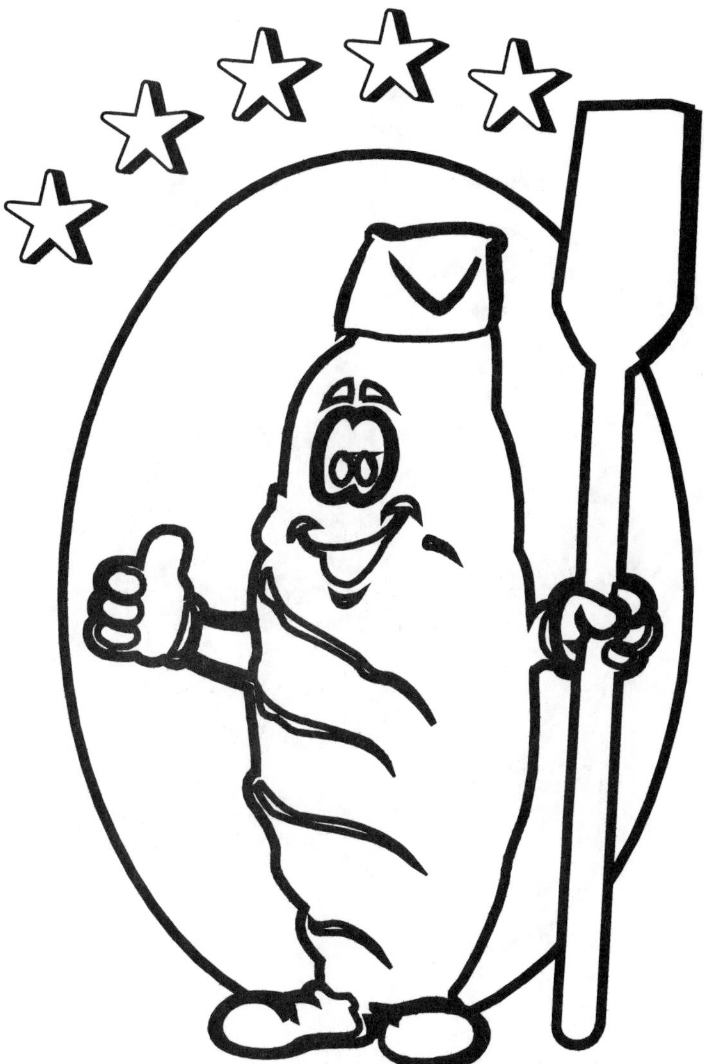

My name is Billy. I'm made out of wheat and oats and lots of other yummy grains. I can help you think better and fight off yucky germs. I can help you sleep, too.

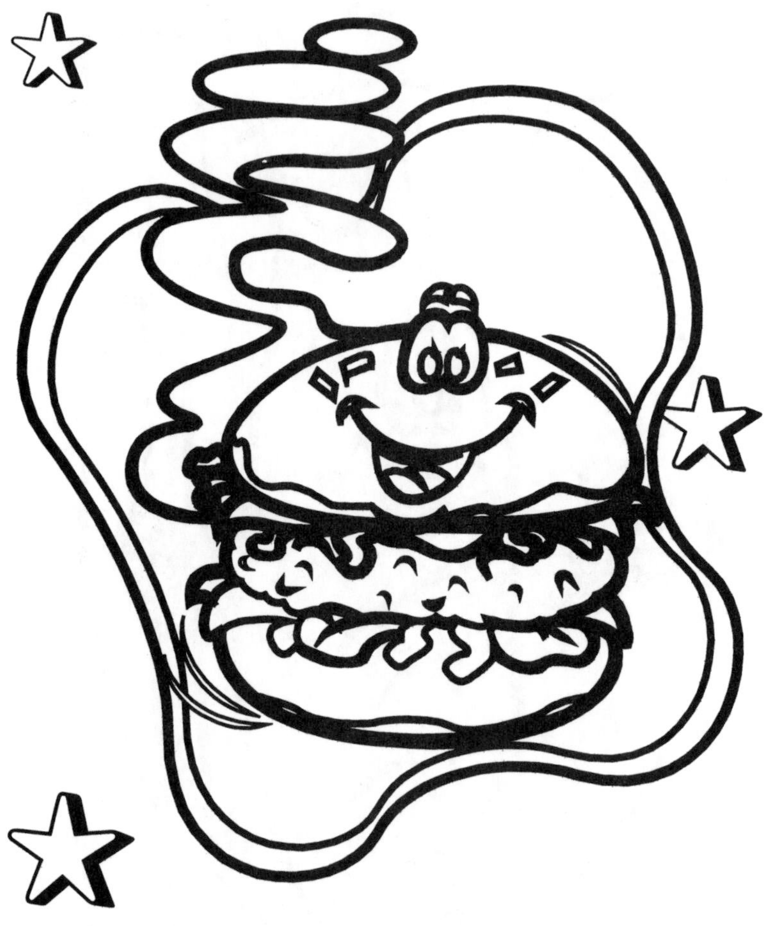

I'm Hannah. I bet you didn't know I can be good *and* be good for you, did you? Well, It's true! I can. My tomatoes can help your muscles grow and help your teeth be strong and healthy, too. What a deal!

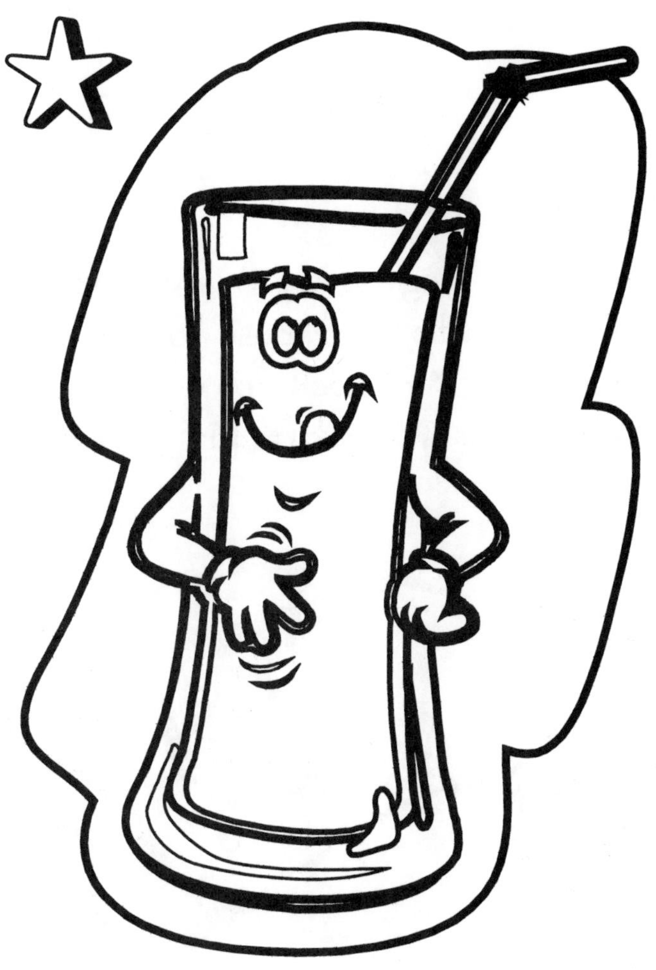

I'm Wendy Water. I'm a real star. When you drink me I will make all of the parts of your body work better! So, be sure to drink me lots every single day.

And I am Super Veggie. My friends and I are coming soon to your house to help you become a Super Kid! Look for us on your table. We won't even get mad if you bite us.

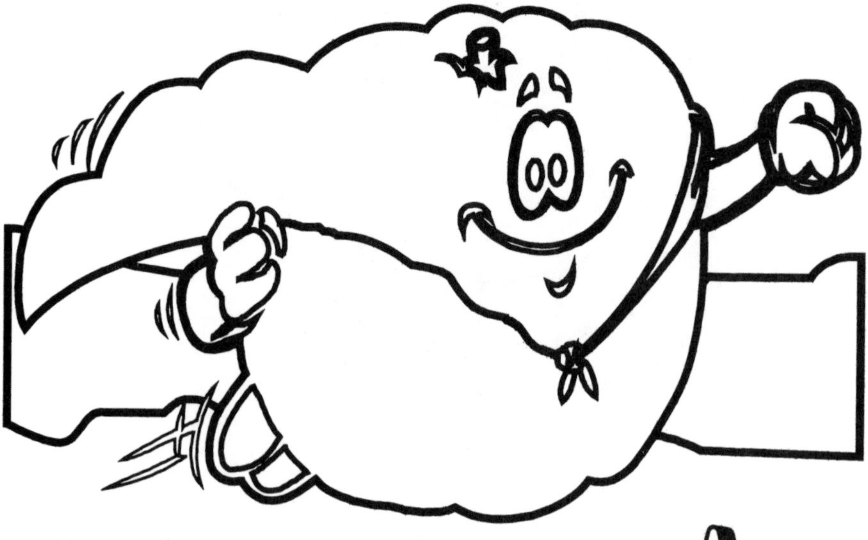

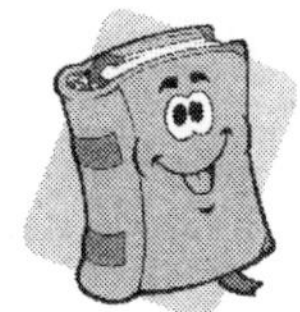

Bibliography

Braly, James, M.D. *Dr. Braly's Food Allergy & Nutrition Revolution*. New Canaan, CT: Keats Publishing, Inc., 1992.

Galland, Leo, M.D., and Dian Dincin Buchman, Ph.D. *Superimmunity for Kids*. New York, NY: Copestone Press, Inc., 1988.

Gislason, Stephen J., M.D. *Core Diet For Kids*. Vancouver, BC: PerSona Audiovisual Productions, 1989.

Golan, Ralph, M.D. *Optimal Wellness*. New York, NY: Ballantine Books, 1995.

Green, Nancy Sokol. *Poisoning Our Children*. Chicago, IL: Noble Press Inc., 1991.

Lansky, Vicki. *Feed Me! I'm Yours*. New York, NY: Bantam Books, 1974.

Larson, Gena. *Better Food for Better Babies and Their Families*. New Canaan, CT: Keats Publishing, Inc., 1972.

McDonald, Linda. *Instant Baby Food.* South Pasadena, CA: Oaklawn Press, Inc., 1975.

Mendelsohn, Robert S., M.D. *How to Raise a Healthy Child ... in Spite of Your Doctor*. New York, NY: Ballantine Books, 1984.

Miller, Dr. Bruce B. *Optimal Nutrition for Healthy Children.* Dallas, TX: Bruce Miller Enterprises, Inc., 1994.

Mindell, Dr. Earl R. Ph., Ph.D. *Parents' Nutrition Bible*. Carson, CA: Hay House, Inc., 1992.

Percival, Mark, D.C., N.D. *The Health Coach Presents Infant Nutrition.* New Hambur, ON: Health Coach Systems International Inc., 1994.

Powers, Hugh, M.D. and James Presley. *Food Power: Nutrition and Your Child's Behavior*. New York, NY: St. Martin's Press, 1978.

Samuels, Mike, M.D. and Nancy Samuels. *The Well Baby Book.* New York, NY: Simon & Schuster, 1991.

Schmidt, Dr. Michael A. *Childhood Ear Infections*. Berkeley, CA: North Atlantic Books, 1990.

Venolia, Carol. *Healing Environments*. Berkeley, CA: Celestial Arts, 1988.

Weber, Marcea. *Encyclopedia of Natural Health and Healing for Children*. Rocklin, CA: Prima Publishing, 1992.

Zand, Janet, LAc, OMD, Rachel Walton, RN, and Bob Rountree, M.D. *Smart Medicine for a Healthier Child.* Garden City Park, NY: Avery Publishing Group, 1994.

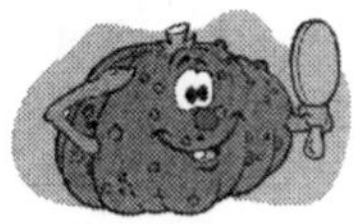

Index

D

E

F

G

H

N

O

P

Q

R

S

T

U

V

W

X

Y

Z

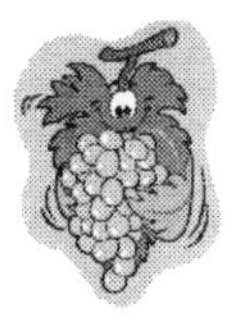

AUTHOR

Cheryl Townsley is the founder of Lifestyle for Health, a company dedicated to helping people restore their total health to its full God-given potential. Cheryl has been a keynote speaker for national seminars, conferences and trade associations. She has been featured on hundreds of national and international television and radio programs.

Cheryl is known for her insight and humor, evident as she provides practical strategies to restore health. All, from individuals to whole families, will find opportunity to step into health with hope and encouragement with Cheryl. Since 1991, Cheryl has published an international, bimonthly newsletter: the *Lifestyle for Health Newsletter*. In addition she has published six books: *Food Smart!*, *Lifestyle for Health Cookbook*, *Meals in 30 Minutes*, *Kid Smart!*, *Return to Paradise* and *Cleansing Made Simple*.

Cheryl resides in Denver, Colorado, with her husband, Forest, and their daughter, Anna.

more about. . .

Dinner!

Software to Help Busy People Make Great Meals in Minutes

- **Tasty, Lowfat Recipes and Menu Plans.** Dinner! comes with all the recipes from Cookbook for the 90s, a collection of tasty, lowfat recipes that are quick and easy, too.

- **Add-On Cookbooks on Disk**: Get more recipes and menu plans with these Cookbooks on Disk:

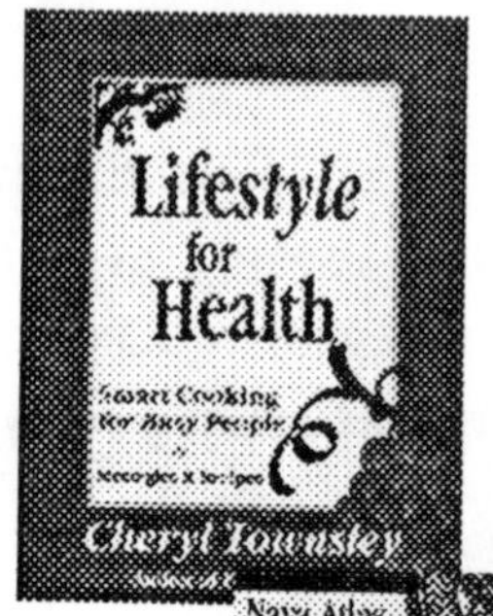

Lifestyle for Health **$14.95**
by Cheryl Townsley
Natural and whole foods collection with 180 recipes and 8 weekly menu plans.

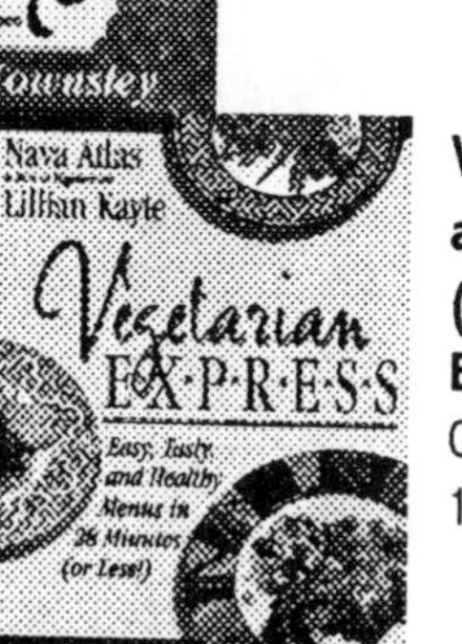

Vegetarian Express: Easy Tasty, and Healthy Menus in 28 Minutes (or Less!) **$15.95**
By Nava Atlas and Lillian Kayte
Creative and quick vegetarian cooking with 150 recipes and 70 dinner menus.

- **Nutritional Information:** See the nutritional content of menu plans, recipes and ingredients.

- **Add and Organize Your Own Recipes:** Nutritional content is calculated automatically

System Requirements

Windows:
386 IBM compatible PC or better
4 MB RAM
Windows 3.1 or higher
7 MB hard drive space

Macintosh
68020 processor or better
4 MB RAM
System 7 or higher
7 MB hard drive space

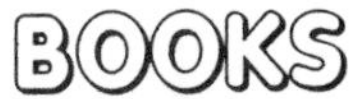

Lifestyle for Health Cookbook

by Cheryl Townsley

Delicious health food including: 8 weeks of menus and grocery lists, over 180 recipes with nutritional analysis, alternatives for sugar, white flour, fat, salt and dairy, many references and much more. Wire spiral bound $24.00

Revised Meals in 30 Minutes

by Cheryl Townsley

Learn the best foods your body needs to maintain weight, mood and energy balance. Tasty recipes help you cook once and eat many times. Recommended supplements for busy people and a section on making cooking fun make this book a winner. $15.00

Cookbook Special —

Set of both cookbooks $35.00

Kid Smart!

by Cheryl Townsley

Information, strategies and recipes to help transition any person — child or adult — from the average American diet to a healthier diet. Includes information on natural alternatives to antibiotics and solutions for common ailments.$15.00

Food Smart!

by Cheryl Townsley

Cheryl shares her story from her suicide attempt and near death through her journey back to health. Learn how to become emotionally and mentally, as well as physically, healthy. A great story that provides practical insight, along with practical helps to health. $14.00

Get Smart Special —

Get both *Kid Smart!* and *Food Smart!* for one great price! $25.00

Cleansing made simple

by Cheryl Townsley

This easy–to–read book explains how the body works, hidden sources of toxins and the basics of cleansing. One chapter is dedicated to cleansing and children. Resources, how–to's and recommendations are provided. $8.00

Return to Paradise

by Cheryl Townsley

Is your life scattered with tiredness and sickness? Are you living a life of lack and dissatisfaction? *Return to Paradise* brings insight on these modern-day death grips. God created a beautiful garden for mankind. Adam and Eve had perfect health, perfect provision and God–given purpose ... You can too! $12.00

Understanding Fats & Oils

by Michael Murray, N.D., and Jade Beutler, R.R.T., R.C.P.

This is the best book I have read to help you understand the differences between good and bad fats. Has recipes for flaxseed oil. $5.00

NEWSLETTER

Lifestyle for Health

12 pages of nutritional information, recipes, health updates, new product reviews and a touch of humor. 6 issues/year $16.00

SOFTWARE

Dinner! and Lifestyle for Health Cookbook

This computer software is easy to use and a real time saver! It includes 16 weeks of menus, recipes, grocery lists and nutritional charts — plus the capability to add and analyze your own recipes.

Available for IBM & Macintosh computers. System requirements — 386 or higher IBM compatible PC • 4MB RAM • Microsoft Windows 3.1 or higher • requires 7.5 MB hard drive space

Add $4.00 shipping/handling per item to order instead of 15%.

Please specify MAC or IBM PC on order form. $65.00

SUPPLEMENTS

MannaCleanse

Our favorite daily cleanse in caplet form. $38.00

Concentrace Mineral Drops

The best value and source for mineral supplementation we have found. $10.50

Barlean's Flax Oil

12 oz. $12.00

Digest-A-Meal Enzymes

$26.00

Total Flora Support

Friendly probiotic support. $26.00

Phyt-Aloe

Plant phytochemicals and antioxidant support for a strong immune system. $38.00

Phyto-Bears

Phyt-Aloe in a gummy-bear form, a real favorite with kids of all ages!
$19.50

Plus

Endocrine, adrenal and hormone system support. $38.00

Sport

Supports lean tissue development and muscle recovery after sports workouts. $35.00

Man-Aloe

Supports cellular communication. $38.00

Metabolic Profile #1

Multi-Vitamin $44.00

Metabolic Profile #2

Multi-Vitamin $44.00

Metabolic Profile #3

Multi-Vitamin $44.00

Kyo-Green

Our favorite greens food drink. $28.00

All prices subject to change.

ORDER FORM

ITEM NAME	QTY.	PRICE	TOTAL

Subtotal	
Shipping & Handling — add 15%	
Tax (CO residents 3.8%)	
Total	

For fastest service fax your credit card order to (303) 794–1449

Charge to my ❑ VISA or ❑ MASTERCARD

Credit Card # ____________________ Exp. Date __________

Authorization Signature ______________________________

Name ______________________________

Address ______________________________

City ____________________ State ______ Zip ____________

Day Phone (   ) ______________________________

Send check or money order to:
Lifestyle for Health
P.O. Box 3871
Littleton, CO 80161
(303) 794–4477

ORDER FORM

ITEM NAME	QTY.	PRICE	TOTAL

For fastest service fax your credit card order to (303) 794–1449

Charge to my ❑ VISA or ❑ MASTERCARD

Credit Card # ____________ Exp. Date ________

Authorization Signature ____________

Name ____________

Address ____________

City ________ State ______ Zip ______

Day Phone (   ) ____________

Subtotal	
Shipping & Handling — add 15%	
Tax (CO residents 3.8%)	
Total	

Send check or money order to:
Lifestyle for Health
P.O. Box 3871
Littleton, CO 80161
(303) 794–4477